"Combines a rounded and psychologically nuanced approach v strategies for supporting a person with dementia who is experiencing distressing behaviours. By encouraging the reader to put themselves in the shoes of the person, the book really gets to the heart of behaviours that challenge. Highly recommended for frontline staff supporting people with dementia."

– *Bernadine McCrory, Alzheimer's Society (Country Director – Northern Ireland), UK*

"A fantastic resource for professional and family carers of people with dementia! Part 1 is a most accessible overview of the dementias and the brain that would also interest people with an early diagnosis. Part 2 is a treasure trove of materials that will facilitate training, empower carers and improve quality of life."

– *Reinhard Guss, Dementia Workstream Lead, Faculty of the Psychology of Older People, British Psychological Society, UK*

"'A complicated topic made simple.' Frances cleverly combines theory with practical insights and examples about the behaviours that challenge people living with dementia. This book is an impartation from a woman who is a credible expert in this subject and it will challenge and encourage you to change the way you deliver care."

– *Eleanor Ross, MBE, Assistant Director Nursing, HSC Public Health Agency, UK*

"Frances Duffy has presented us with a very clearly written account of a relatively new biopsychosocial model for understanding and fulfilling the needs of people with dementia. The CLEAR framework has recently been cited as an example of good practice in the British Psychological Society's briefing paper on treatments for Behaviours that challenge.

CLEAR is an example of one of the new and exciting generations of nonpharmacological interventions, although its use of Behavioural charts provide it with an USP that makes it stand out from the others. In terms of the book itself, it provides a good account of the background to the needs of people with dementia, and the model is well illustrated with helpful examples of case studies."

– *Ian A. James (PhD., MSc., BSc., C.Psychol) Trust Lead Challenging Behaviour Consultant Clinical Psychologist, UK*

"CLEAR builds the insight and competency of caregivers and professionals by enabling them to time-travel into the lives of people living with dementia, with compassion.

It empowers understanding of the behavioural and psychological symptoms of dementia such as agitation, depression, apathy, repetitive questioning, psychosis, aggression, wandering and sleep problems.

The complexity of these symptoms means that there is no 'one size fits all solution' and the CLEAR model provides the paradigm shift required to tailor support.

This is a must read for all in health care settings and in the community."

– *Linda Robinson, Chief Executive Age NI*

CLEAR DEMENTIA CARE©

of related interest

Understanding Behaviour in Dementia that Challenges, Second Edition
A Guide to Assessment and Treatment
Ian Andrew James and Louisa Jackman
ISBN 978 1 78592 264 0
eISBN 978 1 78450 551 6

Person-Centred Dementia Care, Second Edition
Making Services Better with the VIPS Framework
Dawn Brooker and Isabelle Latham
ISBN 978 1 84905 666 3
eISBN 978 1 78450 170 9

The Pool Activity Level (PAL) Instrument for Occupational Profiling
A Practical Resource for Carers of People with Cognitive Impairment, Fourth Edition
Jackie Pool
Part of the University of Bradford Dementia Good Practice Guides series
ISBN 978 1 84905 221 4
eISBN 978 0 85700 463 5

Adaptive Interaction and Dementia
How to Communicate without Speech
Dr Maggie Ellis and Professor Arlene Astell,
Illustrated by Suzanne Scott
ISBN 978 178592 197 1
eISBN 978 1 78450 471 7

CLEAR DEMENTIA CARE ©

A Model to
Assess and Address
Unmet Needs

Dr Frances Duffy

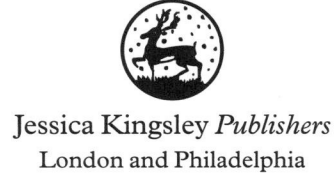

Jessica Kingsley *Publishers*
London and Philadelphia

The CLEAR model is used with kind permission from the Northern Health and Social Care Trust.

First published in 2019
by Jessica Kingsley Publishers
73 Collier Street
London N1 9BE, UK
and
400 Market Street, Suite 400
Philadelphia, PA 19106, USA

www.jkp.com

Copyright © Frances Duffy 2019

All rights reserved. No part of this publication may be reproduced in any material form (including photocopying, storing in any medium by electronic means or transmitting) without the written permission of the copyright owner except in accordance with the provisions of the law or under terms of a licence issued in the UK by the Copyright Licensing Agency Ltd. www.cla.co.uk or in overseas territories by the relevant reproduction rights organisation, for details see www.ifrro.org. Applications for the copyright owner's written permission to reproduce any part of this publication should be addressed to the publisher.

Warning: The doing of an unauthorised act in relation to a copyright work may result in both a civil claim for damages and criminal prosecution.

Library of Congress Cataloging in Publication Data
A CIP catalog record for this book is available from the Library of Congress

British Library Cataloguing in Publication Data
A CIP catalogue record for this book is available from the British Library

ISBN 978 1 78592 276 3
eISBN 978 1 78450 576 9

Printed and bound in Great Britain

> All pages marked with ★ can be photocopied and downloaded at www.jkp.com/voucher for personal use with this program, but may not be reproduced for any other purposes without the permission of the publisher.

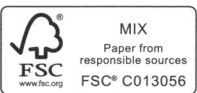

CONTENTS

Acknowledgements — 6

PART 1: UNDERSTANDING DEMENTIA AND BEHAVIOUR — 9

1. Dementia and the Brain — 11
2. Types of Dementia — 19
3. Dementia and Loss — 37
4. Dementia and Sense of Self — 51
5. Understanding Behaviour — 57
6. Recording Behaviour — 69
7. What Do People with Dementia Need? — 75

PART 2: IMPLEMENTING THE CLEAR DEMENTIA CARE© MODEL — 81

8. Domains of CLEAR Dementia Care© — 83
9. The Experience of Carers — 133
10. Supporting Care Staff — 141
11. A Case Example — 147

Appendices — 159
References — 167
Index — 169

ACKNOWLEDGEMENTS

When I think about how I would treat a person with dementia, I think about how I would treat my mother and father, with the endless love, kindness and compassion that they have shown me.

When you are loved and cared for, you can be who you are.

For Roisin, Sorcha and Odhran, whose enthusiasm for life inspires me every day.

CLEAR Dementia Care© was developed in the Northern Health and Social Care Trust Dementia Home Support Team. The successful development is due to the commitment and enthusiasm of Marc Harvey and the team, who consistently work to improve the quality of life for people living with dementia. It is a privilege to work in an innovative and caring team who strive for excellence.

The Northern Health and Social Care Trust offers a CLEAR Dementia Care© training programme aimed at care home staff, and a CLEAR Dementia Care© Train the Trainer programme. For further information please contact CLEAR. DementiaCare@northerntrust.hscni.net

PART 1

UNDERSTANDING DEMENTIA AND BEHAVIOUR

Chapter 1

DEMENTIA AND THE BRAIN

As we get older we gradually do things more slowly. We can't run as fast as we could when we were younger and the way our brain processes information also slows. We become more forgetful and process information less efficiently.

At any age we can have the experience of forgetting where we have put things, such as our glasses or keys, or going into a room and forgetting why we are there. These are normal slips of memory and they increase as we get older. When this happens, it can be frustrating and we attribute it to not paying attention, having too many things to do, being distracted or, as we get older, to "a senior moment". We recognise that as we get older these slips of memory come with the territory, but they don't have a big impact on our ability to carry on with our everyday activities. We just try to take things a bit more slowly, pay attention and not do too many things at the same time.

Some people experience changes in their everyday function which cannot be explained by normal age-related changes. Increasing age also increases the likelihood of developing dementia. Dementia is a term used to describe a number of conditions which lead to progressive changes in the structure of the brain that affect how the brain functions.

These changes can affect how the person thinks, feels, behaves and their ability to complete everyday tasks. To be consistent with a diagnosis of dementia, the difficulties experienced must interfere with social and occupational function or normal activities of daily living. While the risk of dementia increases with age, it is not an inevitable part of ageing.

The Alzheimer's Society Dementia UK Report (Prince *et al.* 2014) estimated that there were 850,000 people living with dementia in the UK in 2014. A person's risk of developing dementia rises from *one in 14* people over the age of 65, to *one in six* people over the age of 80. While most people with dementia are aged over 65 years, dementia can also affect people under 65 years. The Alzheimer Society report estimated that there were over 42,000 people under 65 years with young onset dementia in the UK in 2013. It is estimated that one in three people born in 2015 will develop dementia (Lewis 2015).

Dementia impacts on the person and their family, friends and carers. It is estimated that 38 per cent of the population – 24.6 million people in the UK – have a family member or close friend who is living with dementia (Alzheimer's Research UK).

Dementia is a progressive condition and, while every person is different, Mary's story is example of how things can change.

MARY'S STORY

Mary lives at home with her husband John; they have two children, Jane and Tom. Jane lives close by and visits every week. Tom lives about four hours' drive away and visits once a month. Mary has three grandchildren Sarah (9), Mike (6) and Finn (3) who also visit most weeks with their mum, Jane. Jane's husband Jeff visits frequently. Mary attends her local church on Sunday and has a few close friends in the local community.

Jane visited her mother on Saturday and when they were taking about her brother Tom, Mary said, "Tom never comes to visit anymore". Jane reminded her mum that Tom had visited the weekend before but Mary had no recollection of the visit.

On another visit, Mary got mixed up with her grandchildren's names. She was also less tolerant of the children. When they were playing she asked them to be quite in a tone of voice that seemed cross. This was uncharacteristic of

Mary as she always looked forward to the grandchildren visiting and enjoyed watching them play.

Mary's husband, John, noticed a change in her baking skills. Mary had always been an excellent baker and he looked forward to her weekly batch of scones. They tasted different and he asked her if she had used a different recipe. Mary became cross with John and said if he didn't like her baking he could make his own scones. John was surprised as this was not how Mary would normally speak to him. As the weeks progressed, John noticed that Mary was less able to prepare the dinner which she had always cooked independently. She cooked the potatoes before she put the meat on, which meant that different parts of the dinner were cooked at different times. On another occasion, the potatoes boiled dry and burned the saucepan. She became frustrated and cross and blamed John for distracting her. John began to offer more support with preparing meals which caused some tension and often Mary would tell John that if he thought he could do it better he should do it himself. This was unlike Mary who had always been a mild-mannered, easy-going lady.

When friends came to visit, Mary appeared withdrawn. She was not her usual self and did not contribute much to the conversation. When she did speak sometimes what she said was not connected to the topic of conversation. Her friends seemed puzzled but did not make a fuss. On one occasion, Mary went to the kitchen to make tea. When she had been gone for some time John went to the kitchen to see if she needed help. Mary was sitting at the kitchen table looking at a magazine. She had become distracted and forgotten that she was making tea for visitors.

Mary and John went to the supermarket together to do the weekly shop. John noticed that Mary was not organised during their shop. She would traditionally have prepared a list and systematically walked along each aisle to find the things on her list. Her shopping was more haphazard, she had no list and lifted items that they did not need and failed to buy items that they did need. When paying for the shopping she had difficulty counting the appropriate amount of money. When John offered to help, she became cross and told him he was confusing her.

Mary's story suggests that she is becoming more forgetful and this seems to be having an impact on her daily activities. Is she in the early stages of dementia? Mary may have dementia but there are many other potential causes for changes in function. It is important if you think that you or a family member may have dementia that you speak to your GP. The GP will complete the appropriate tests to ensure that there are no treatable conditions that may be causing the symptoms and, if appropriate, may refer to a specialist service.

Certain medical conditions can cause changes in thinking and behaviour which may appear to be a dementia. The symptoms should improve when the person gets appropriate treatment. Medical conditions that may cause memory problems include:

- Tumors, blood clots, or infections in the brain.
- Some thyroid, kidney, or liver disorders.
- Drinking too much alcohol.
- Head injury, such as a concussion from a fall or accident.
- Medication side effects (National Institute on Aging, n.d.).
- Not eating enough healthy foods (National Institute on Aging, n.d.) or too few vitamins and minerals in a person's body (like vitamin B12).
- Depression.
- Sleep disturbance.

There are many different types of dementia and each type tends to have a characteristic profile and specific early symptoms. This is because, for different types of dementia, different parts of the brain are affected first. As the dementia progresses and damage spreads to more areas of the brain, the symptoms of different types of dementia become more similar.

THE BRAIN

The brain has 100 billion brain cells (neurons). The brain controls all the functions of the body and interprets information coming in from the senses: sight, smell, taste, touch and hearing. Each brain cell connects with many other brain cells to form communication networks. The brain cells communicate with each other, a bit like people talking to each other on phones. Groups of brain cells have specific jobs. Some are involved in thinking, learning and remembering. Others help us to move, taste, see, hear and smell.

To do their job, brain cells need to communicate with each other and store information. Dementia prevents parts of the brain from working. When one part of the brain is not working, the other parts of the brain that are connected to that part don't receive some of the information they need to do their jobs. This is what causes the problems in thinking, feeling and behaviour.

Different parts of the brain are responsible for different functions, although there are many connections between them.

The outermost layer of the brain is the wrinkly cerebral cortex – the grey matter – which is made up of tightly packed brain cells. This is divided into four different lobes: the frontal, parietal, temporal, and occipital lobes. These lobes are each responsible for processing different types of information coming from our senses. There are many complex interactions between each of the lobes and any function is likely to be the responsibility of more than one lobe.

The different parts of the brain are connected through white matter tracts. The white matter can be thought of as the roads inside the brain that link together all the different parts. The white matter allows fast communication between different parts of the brain. Some types of dementia affect the white matter in the brain.

THE FRONTAL LOBE

The frontal lobe, located at the front of the brain, can be thought of as the control centre to the brain and the home of our personality. It enables us to monitor and control our emotions and behaviour so that we do not do or say things that are not appropriate for the particular situation we are in. For example, there are certain things that you might do or say when you are with your friends that you would not do or say when you are with colleagues in work or people you don't know very well. You are more likely to tell friends things about your personal life that you wouldn't tell to strangers. The frontal lobe of the brain helps to keep a check on what we are doing and saying and stop us doing and saying things that are not appropriate.

Damage to the frontal lobe can mean that a person will say things or behave in ways that are not appropriate for the situation. A person with damage to the frontal lobe may say something or do something without thinking about the consequence or the impact this may have on another person. For example, they see a person who is wearing a dress that they do not like. Your frontal lobe stops you from telling the person you don't like the dress because you know that it might hurt their feelings. If you had damage to the frontal lobe you may not be able to stop yourself.

If something happens that makes us feel very cross or angry, the frontal lobe of our brain helps us control how we react. Damage to the frontal lobe may mean that the person is unable to control their behaviour so they may shout and become aggressive.

The frontal lobe is involved when we make decisions, for example about what to eat for lunch or where we want to live. If you ask someone with damage to the frontal lobe what they want for lunch they may not be able to choose. Offering two alternatives can help. Do you want a sandwich or soup? The frontal lobe is also important to help us weigh up the pros and cons of a decision and understand the consequences of that decision. Damage can have serious consequences and the person may make decisions impulsively or make decisions that are risky without considering the consequences; for example, buying an expensive item without considering whether they have enough money to pay for the item or whether they actually need it.

The frontal lobe is involved in planning and organising. Think about planning what to make for dinner. In order to do this, you need to know what the end product will be, for example roast chicken, potatoes and peas followed by apple pie. How do you make the dinner? You need to think about all the things you need and make sure you have them. The final step is the actual cooking, which all needs to be sequenced and timed so that the food is prepared correctly and is ready to be served in the correct order. Our frontal lobe helps us to perform this co-ordinated planning.

If we are hungry and see someone eating, we do not take the food from their plate. Our frontal lobe helps us to control this desire and, instead, ask for our own food or prepare our own food. Similarly, we may feel the urge to urinate when we are at the supermarket. Our frontal lobe facilitates our holding our urine until we get to the bathroom. Our frontal lobe inhibits inappropriate responses such as taking food from someone or going to the toilet in an inappropriate place.

The person may or may not be aware that their behaviour is inappropriate. Some people may be unable to control their behaviour but may also be embarrassed and horrified at what they have done. Others have no awareness that they have done something wrong.

Our personality is formed in the frontal lobe – whether we are a quiet, sociable person, easy going or highly strung. Damage to the frontal lobe can result in a change in personality and also a change in mood.

PARIETAL LOBE

The parietal lobe, located in the middle top part of the brain, integrates sensory information from different parts of the body and processes information from the sense of touch.

The parietal lobe enables us to see where objects are, reach for them and manipulate them. Depth perception enables us to see the world in three dimensions and judge the distances between objects. Damage to the parietal lobe can cause apraxia, which is impairment in planning and making movements. You want to lift a cup, you can see the cup, you have the ability to move your arm but your brain cannot plan the movement to effectively move your arm to reach the accurate location of the cup. Performing all the movements required to get dressed can be very difficult with damage to the parietal lobe. Other activities such as opening a door or brushing your teeth can also be difficult.

The parietal lobe is important for spatial awareness. Damage can cause the person to be clumsy, bump into things or cause other objects to bump into things, for example hitting the curb with your car. To be able to navigate effectively, we need to know where our body is in relation to other things in the environment.

The parietal lobe is also involved with mathematics, reading, writing, drawing and spelling.

TEMPORAL LOBE

The temporal lobe is located in the lower, temple region of the brain. It is responsible for controlling our speech, enabling us to understand what is being said and remember the information that we hear. This is important for engaging in conversation, as we need to understand what has been said, remember what has been said and then respond with what we want to say.

The temporal lobe is also important for processing, interpreting and remembering visual information, such as objects, faces, pictures and scenery.

The temporal lobe is involved in encoding and creating new memories in the brain and storing these memories. These memories can be facts such as remembering that a cat is an animal, or memories for specific events, for example that your friend visited on Wednesday and brought a bunch of flowers.

The temporal lobe is necessary to navigate spatially. With damage to the temporal lobe, a person can get lost because their brain is unable to process, spatially, where they have been and where they are going.

OCCIPITAL LOBE

The occipital lobe is important to enable understanding and making sense of what your eyes are seeing. The occipital lobe is involved in visuospatial processing, recognition that objects are moving and recognising colours. Damage to the occipital lobe can cause visual hallucinations (seeing things that are not there) and visual illusions (distorted perceptions such as objects appearing bigger or smaller than they actually are, objects lacking colour or objects having abnormal colouring).

Chapter 2

TYPES OF DEMENTIA

There are over a hundred different types of dementia. The most common is Alzheimer's disease (62%), vascular dementia (17%), Lewy body dementia (4%), fronto-temporal dementia (2%) and mixed Alzheimer's and vascular dementia (10%). Over 100 other dementias account for the remaining 3 per cent of cases (Prince *et al.* 2014).

How dementia affects the brain and the person will depend on the type of dementia, what stage the dementia is at and a variety of other factors, including physical health, the environment and supports the person has access to. Dementia is a progressive condition, which means that over time the ability to think and communicate gets worse and there is increased dependence on other people to meet everyday needs. While this presents a significant challenge to the person and their family, a better understanding of dementia can have a very positive impact on wellbeing.

When caring for a person with dementia, it is important to know what type of dementia they have because this will provide information on what their areas of strength and weakness are likely to be. This can also help with making decisions about how best to support the person, using their strengths to help compensate for areas of weakness.

ALZHEIMER'S DISEASE

Alzheimer's disease is the most common type of dementia and accounts for about 62 per cent of cases diagnosed (Prince *et al.* 2014). Alzheimer's disease destroys brain cells. Two proteins which occur naturally in the brain, amyloid and tau, become abnormal and begin to malfunction. Plaques and tangles form, which kill the brain cells. (Plaques are deposits of beta amyloid which stick together and form clumps around dead brain cells, stopping the cells from sending messages to each other. Tangles are twisted fibres found inside brain cells which are made from the protein tau. Tangles stop the transport of nutrients and other important substances between brain cells.) Gaps develop when brain cells die and the brain shrinks. People with Alzheimer's disease also have a reduction of a chemical in the brain called acetylcholine, which acts as a messenger taking information from one brain cell to other brain cells. A reduction in acetylcholine means that information is not being transmitted and the brain cells cannot communicate effectively with each other.

Alzheimer's disease causes impairment in the person's ability to think, remember, speak and make decisions. It is progressive, which means that as more parts of the brain are damaged, more symptoms develop. The symptoms also become more severe.

Even within Alzheimer's disease there are different types. The type of Alzheimer's disease depends on the part of the brain that is damaged first. As the dementia progresses, damage spreads to all areas of the brain and the different types become similar.

AMNESIC ALZHEIMER'S DISEASE

Amnesic Alzheimer's disease is the most common type. In the early stages, the damage is in the hippocampus, part of the temporal lobe of the brain. This part of the brain is essential to make new memories. The first symptoms are problems with memory. The person is likely to forget recent conversations, ask the same question many times and become disorientated, even in familiar places. They may also have difficulty finding words in conversation. Memories from the past remain intact until the later stages.

ATYPICAL ALZHEIMER'S DISEASE

In the other types of Alzheimer's disease, the damage caused by plaques and tangles is the same, but the first part of the brain affected is not the hippocampus and so the earliest symptoms are not memory loss. Atypical Alzheimer's disease is more common in people diagnosed when they are aged under 65 years with early onset Alzheimer's disease.

POSTERIOR CORTICAL ATROPHY

Posterior cortical atrophy (PCA) occurs when there is damage to areas at the back and upper-rear of the brain, the occipital and parietal lobes. These are the areas that process visual information and spatial awareness. This means that the early symptoms of PCA are usually problems identifying what objects are or reading. Problems with going up and down stairs can also occur because there is impairment in the ability to judge distances. The person can become uncoordinated and find it difficult to get dressed. This is not a problem with eyesight because the impairment occurs even if the eyes are healthy.

The first symptoms of PCA tend to occur when people are in their mid-50s or early 60s. The first signs are often subtle and so it may be some time before a formal diagnosis is made. Initially, people with PCA tend to have a relatively well-preserved memory.

LOPOGENIC PROGRESSIVE APHASIA

Logopenic progressive aphasia involves damage to the areas in the left side of the brain, the temporal and parietal lobes. These areas are involved in producing language. The first symptoms occur in speech. The person's speech becomes laboured with long pauses. They find it difficult to repeat a sentence and there is difficulty finding the right word in conversation.

DYSEXECUTIVE ALZHEIMER'S DISEASE

Dysexecutive Alzheimer's disease involves damage to the frontal lobe of the brain. The symptoms include problems with planning and decision making. The person may also behave in ways that are socially inappropriate or it may appear that they do not care about the feelings of others.

SYMPTOMS OF AMNESIC ALZHEIMER'S DISEASE

There are some common symptoms of amnesic Alzheimer's disease, but it is important to remember that everyone is unique. Two people with Alzheimer's disease are unlikely to experience the condition in exactly the same way.

The symptoms are generally mild to start with, but they get worse over time and start to interfere with daily life. Early symptoms include:

- Regularly misplacing items such as keys, glasses and wallet or putting them in odd places.
- Difficulty recalling recent events and conversations.
- Becoming increasingly repetitive, for example asking the same questions multiple times.
- Difficulty learning new information, for example how to use a new microwave or TV remote.
- Struggling to find the right word in a conversation or forgetting someone's name.
- Finding it hard to follow conversations or TV programmes.
- Getting lost in a familiar place.
- Forgetting appointments, birthdays or anniversaries.
- Getting confused with money and forgetting to pay bills.
- Difficulty shopping or preparing meals.
- Being less able to plan, problem solve, organise and think logically.

- Taking longer to complete normal daily tasks.

- Exhibiting changes in personality or behaviour.

- Loss of enthusiasm for previously enjoyed hobbies and activities.

- Becoming more withdrawn.

- Mood swings – feeling sad and angry or scared and frustrated.

Memory for events that happened a long time ago is often unaffected in the early stages.

Dementia gets worse over time, but the speed of decline varies from person to person. As the dementia progresses, it begins to interfere with more activities of daily living.

- Memory for events that happened before the dementia begin to decline.

- There is disorientation and confusion about the time and place.

- The ability to make decisions gets worse.

- Communication becomes more difficult. There are problems with speaking, understanding and following a conversation, and with reading and writing.

- There is difficulty recognising household objects, familiar faces and places.

- Day-to-day tasks become harder, for example using a TV remote control, phone or kitchen appliances.

- There may be difficulty finding an object even when it is right in front of the person, for example finding keys that are sitting on the kitchen table.

- Changes in sleep patterns often occur – the person may be up more in the night.

- Some people become sad, depressed or frustrated about the challenges they face.

- Anxiety is also common and the person may become fearful or suspicious.

- The person may experience hallucinations, where they may see things or people that are not there.

- Some people experience delusions where they start to believe things that are not true.

- People may become increasingly unsteady on their feet and are at greater risk of falling.

- Daily activities like dressing, using the toilet and eating become more difficult.

- The person may become lost in familiar places.

- The person may leave their home at night.

- They may behave inappropriately, for example going outdoors in nightwear.

- They may be neglectful of hygiene or eating.

In the later stages of Alzheimer's disease, the person may appear to be much less aware of what is happening around them. They may have difficulties eating and walking, and become increasingly frail. Eventually, the person will need help with all their daily activities.

VASCULAR DEMENTIA

Vascular dementia is the second most common type of dementia in people aged over 65 years and accounts for around 17 per cent of cases (Prince *et al.* 2014). Vascular dementia in people aged under the age of 65 is comparatively rare.

Vascular dementia is an umbrella term for a group of conditions caused by different types of vascular brain injury which cause problems with blood circulation to the brain. To be healthy and function properly, brain cells need a constant supply of blood to bring oxygen and nutrients. Blood is delivered to the brain through a network of vessels called the vascular system. If the vascular system within the brain becomes damaged and blood cannot reach the brain cells, the cells will eventually die. This happens when blood vessels leak or become blocked.

There are different types of vascular dementia. The difference between each type depends on what has caused the damage in the brain, and which part of the brain has been damaged. The two main types are caused by stroke or by small vessel disease.

STROKE-RELATED OR MULTI-INFARCT DEMENTIA

When any part of the body is deprived of blood it can die. This is called an infarct. When this happens in an area of the brain it is called a stroke. A stroke is usually the result of a burst blood vessel which bleeds (known as haemorrhagic stroke) or a blood vessel in the brain becomes narrowed and is blocked by a clot (known as an ischemic stroke). The clot may have formed in the brain, or it may have formed in the heart and been carried to the brain if someone has heart disease.

Not everyone who has a stroke will develop vascular dementia, but a person who has a stroke is at increased risk of having further strokes. Over time, these strokes build up causing the symptoms of vascular dementia.

The location of the damage determines the nature of impairments observed, leading to great variety in symptoms of a stroke. If the area affected is responsible for movement of an arm or leg, paralysis might occur. If it is responsible for speech, the person might have problems communicating.

SUB-CORTICAL VASCULAR DEMENTIA

This type of dementia, also known as small vessel disease is caused by damage to tiny blood vessels that lie deep in the brain. Years of high blood pressure can result in narrowing of the vessels, which reduces blood flow or can even stop blood flow to the area of the brain supplied by these vessels. These narrower vessels also need higher blood pressure to push blood adequately through them. This higher blood pressure contributes to a vicious cycle, with further blood vessel damage occurring. It's like breathing through a straw – you can do it but it is exhausting and not very effective. The reduced or lack of blood flow to areas of the brain causes the brain cells to die. High blood pressure and diabetes mellitus are risk factors for small vessel disease.

SYMPTOMS

Vascular dementia affects different people in different ways and the speed of the progression varies from person to person. Stroke-related vascular dementia often follows a "stepped" progression, with symptoms remaining at a constant level for a time and then suddenly deteriorating. This is because each additional stroke causes further damage to the brain. As a consequence, there can be rapid onset of changes in thinking, skills or behaviour.

The symptoms depend on the location of the stroke and what brain functions are affected by the damage. Subcortical vascular dementia may occasionally follow this stepped progression, but more often symptoms get worse gradually.

Symptoms can include:

- Gait disturbance with difficulty walking, unsteadiness and increased risk of falls.

- Clumsiness.

- Incontinence because the brain registers the message to pass urine either too late or not at all and the person cannot get to the toilet in time.

- Lack of facial expression.

- Speech difficulties.

- Difficulty with concentration and following a conversation.

- Difficulty with planning, reasoning and judgement.

- Memory problems, but reminding may help because the difficulty is with retrieving information from memory.

- Slower speed of thinking.

- Getting lost.

- Visual misperceptions, for example seeing a rug on the floor as a pond.

- Changes in behaviour, such as restlessness.

- Depression and anxiety.

- Mood swings, laughing or crying for no apparent reason (emotional lability).

- Hallucinations – seeing or hearing things that aren't there.

- Delusions – believing things that are not true.

As the dementia progresses the symptoms get worse:

- More severe confusion and disorientation.
- Reasoning and communication are more impaired.
- Memory gets worse.
- The person will need more support with day-to-day activities such as cooking or cleaning.

In the later stages, the person may become much less aware of what is happening around them. They may have difficulties walking or eating without help, and become increasingly frail. Eventually, the person will need help with all their daily activities.

LEWY BODY DEMENTIA

Lewy body dementia accounts for around 4 per cent of people diagnosed with dementia (Prince *et al.* 2014) and is more common in people over the age of 65 years. It is a progressive condition where the symptoms gradually get worse over time. Lewy bodies are tiny abnormal deposits of a protein (alpha-synuclein) that appear in brain cells. This damages the way the brain cells work and communicate with each other. The lewy bodies are associated with damage to the substantia nigra, a subcortical region of the brain. Brain cells in the substantia nigra produce the chemical messenger dopamine. Dopamine sends signals between the substantia nigra and the basal ganglia in the brain. These signals are important for movement. Disruption of these signals affects movement and balance. Lewy bodies are also associated with damage to the brain cells in the basal forebrain which produce acetylcholine. This damage is associated with impaired thinking and perception and changes in behaviour.

SYMPTOMS

Lewy body dementia can cause fluctuation in ability from moment to moment, hour to hour, day to day or week to week. The person may stare into space for a long time or have periods when they find it difficult to have a conversation. At other times they may be able to pay attention to what you are saying and speak very well. This can be very confusing for carers as the person's ability changes. Carers can find it hard to understand why the person can engage in an activity on one occasion but not another. A person with Lewy body dementia may not fit many people's perception of someone with dementia. It could be assumed that the person is "just being difficult" because they could engage or do an activity earlier but "do not want to" do it now. It is important to understand that they have no control over their fluctuating ability. It is part of the dementia.

Symptoms include:

- Problems with attention, concentration and alertness.

- Brief episodes of unexplained confusion.

- Disorientation about the time or where they are.

- Forgetting recent events (but reminding the person can help them to remember).

- Difficulty with speech, finding words or following a conversation.

- Problems with planning, organising and problem solving.

- Difficulty making decisions. If you ask the person what they want for breakfast they may not be able to make a decision. Offering a choice, say toast or porridge, will help.

- Lack of insight into their difficulties.

- Visuospatial difficulty, for example problems with finding their way around, completing visual tasks, judging depth, distance and seeing objects in three dimensions.

- Visual misperceptions, for example the person can mistake a shadow or a coat on a hanger for a person. This could be frightening if they believe someone is in their room.

- Vivid visual hallucinations – seeing things that are not there. These are commonly of people or animals and they can frighten the person and cause distress.

- Auditory hallucinations – hearing sounds that are not real, such as a knocking sound or footsteps. The person may believe someone is knocking on their door or window or someone is walking around in their room.

- Olfactory ("tasting") or tactile ("feeling") hallucinations are less common but can sometimes occur.

- Delusions – believing something that is not true. Hallucinations and visual misperceptions may explain why people experience delusions. The person may believe that someone is out to get them, that there are strangers in their own room, or that their wife/husband is having an affair or has been replaced by an identical imposter. The person and those who care for them can find these delusions very distressing.

- Movement problems can include stooped posture, shuffling gait, reduced arm swing, stiff or rigid movement, unsteadiness and a tendency to fall, slowness of movement (bradykinesia) and tremor.

- The person may fall asleep very easily during the day, but have restless, disturbed sleep at night. Sleep issues are common in dementia but there is a specific sleep condition called REM Sleep Disorder that appears to affect people with Lewy body dementia. This entails movement, hitting out or yelling at night as the person acts out their dreams. This can be distressing for carers.

- Changes in mood. In some cases, there can be depression.

- They may also have a blank facial expression, which can make it more difficult to interpret how they are feeling.

When caring for someone with Lewy body dementia, it is important to be as flexible as possible, as many of the symptoms will vary over time. Anti-psychotic medication is especially harmful for people with Lewy body dementia.

FRONTOTEMPORAL DEMENTIA

Frontotemporal dementia (FTD) accounts for approximately 2 per cent of cases of dementia (Prince *et al.* 2014) and is more common in younger people in their 50s and 60s. It is caused by abnormally forming proteins including tau and TDP-43, which damage brain cells in the frontal and temporal lobes. Some of the chemical messengers that transmit signals between nerve cells are also lost.

TYPES OF FRONTOTEMPORAL DEMENTIA

The symptoms of FTD dementia vary depending on which areas of the frontal and temporal lobes are damaged first. There are three main types:

- Behavioural variant frontal-temporal dementia.
- Primary progressive aphasias and semantic dementia.
- Motor variants of FTD.

Behavioural variant frontotemporal dementia

This is the most common type of FTD. The initial symptoms include changes in behaviour and personality:

- Behaving inappropriately and losing normal inhibitions.
- Making tactless or inappropriate comments about someone's appearance or other people's misfortune.
- Behaving in a sexual manner in public places.
- Being more extrovert than before.
- Acting more impulsively, for example spending excessive amounts of money.
- Becoming less interested in things and having less motivation to do things.
- Needing prompting to do routine activities
- Paying less attention to personal hygiene and dress.

- Loss of sympathy or empathy and becoming less concerned with the needs of others. This can make the person appear selfish and unfeeling.

- Interacting less with people and withdrawing from social activities.

- Loss of warmth in social interaction.

- Repetitive in behaviour.

- Being rigid and inflexible in the way they do things or having to stick to routines.

- Collecting or hoarding things.

- Changes in the types of food eaten, such as sweet foods.

- Not knowing when to stop eating, drinking alcohol or smoking.

- Being unaware of their problems and lacking insight into what is happening to them.

- Problems in planning, organisation, making decisions or solving problems.

- Difficulty concentrating on one thing and easily distracted.

- Difficulty finding the right word in conversation or understanding what other people are saying.

In the early stages of behavioural variant FTD, memory is relatively preserved. As the dementia progresses, there is decline across all cognitive functions.

PRIMARY PROGRESSIVE APHASIA

Primary progressive aphasia (PPA) consists of semantic dementia and progressive non-fluent aphasia and causes impairment in language function.

Semantic dementia

In semantic dementia, speech is fluent but vocabulary is impaired. Symptoms include:

- Talking about things in a vague manner.

- Difficulty finding a word, saying "the thing you sit on" instead of chair, or using the category instead of the specific name, saying "animal" instead of "dog".

- Difficulty understanding what other people are saying. When asked, would you like toast the person may reply, "What is toast?"

- Difficulty recognising familiar people and common objects.

- Problems with reading.

- Problems with spelling.

Progressive non-fluent aphasia

In progressive non-fluent aphasia, speech is slow and hesitant and may seem effortful; the person may seem to stutter before they can get the right word out. Symptoms include:

- Difficulty finding the right word.

- Pronouncing words incorrectly, for example "aminal" instead of "animal".

- Saying the opposite word to the one they mean to say.

- Telegraphic speech, for example "went shop" instead of "we went to the shop".

- Difficulty understanding complex sentences but able to understand single words.

- Problems with reading.

- Problems with spelling.

In the early stages of PPA, memory and other cognitive functions are relatively intact. As the dementia progresses, there is decline across all cognitive functions.

MOTOR VARIANT FRONTOTEMPORAL DEMENTIA

There are three subtypes of motor variant FTD: corticobasal syndrome (CBS), progressive supranuclear palsy (PSP) and FTD with motor neurone disease (FTD MND).

Corticobasal syndrome CBS

The first symptoms affect movement and usually start on one side of the body. Symptoms usually affect the hand or arm first but it can be the leg and include:

- Clumsiness.
- Slowness of movements (bradykinesia).
- Stiffness and rigidity.
- Shaking (tremors) and spasms (dystonia).
- Loss of feeling.
- Feeling like the limb doesn't belong (an "alien" limb).
- Loss of balance and co-ordination.
- Inability to do complex actions with the hands (limb apraxia), for example difficulty opening a door, operating the television remote, or using kitchen tools.
- Difficulty with speech.
- Slow and slurred speech.

As the dementia progresses, problems spread to both sides of the body and other limbs and symptoms include:

- Memory impairment.
- Problems with language.
- Problems carrying out tasks that require planning or thinking ahead.
- Problems coping with sudden and unexpected situations.
- Difficulty with simple mathematical calculations, such as adding or subtracting.
- Difficulty seeing things, or knowing where they are located.
- Difficulty orienting in space, bumping into things.
- Personality changes, such as becoming apathetic, irritable, agitated or anxious.
- Difficulty swallowing.

Progressive supranuclear palsy (PSP)

Symptoms include:

- Difficulty walking.
- Balance problems.
- Recurrent falls.
- Slow movements.
- Stiffness of the muscles, particularly the neck and trunk muscles.
- Slow speed of thinking.
- Difficulty moving the eyes up and down (ophthalmoplegia). This may not be noticed by the person themselves or their family but will be apparent on medical examination.
- Depression and apathy.

Later on, symptoms include:

- Change in personality.
- Slurring of speech.
- Difficulty swallowing.
- Laughing or crying at inappropriate times (emotional lability).
- Problems with planning, reasoning and problem solving.
- Problems with memory.

Motor neurone disease

Motor neurone disease (MND) is a disorder of the nerves that control the body's motor function. It affects the nerves that go to the muscles in the arms and legs, and those that control speech and swallow.

Symptoms can include:

- Wasting and weakness of muscles.
- Twitching of muscles (fasciculations).
- Stiffness of muscles.
- Problems with articulation, making speech sound slurred (dysarthria).
- Problems with swallowing (dysphagia).

Later in the disease, problems with breathing can develop.

As FTD progresses, the differences between the three types become much less obvious. People with the behavioural variant tend to develop language problems as their condition progresses and they may eventually lose all speech. Similarly, a person with a language variant of FTD will tend to develop the behavioural problems typical of behavioural variant FTD.

MIXED DEMENTIA

Mixed dementia is characterised by the hallmark features of more than one cause of dementia, most commonly Alzheimer's dementia combined with vascular dementia.

OTHER DEMENTIAS

There are many other types of dementia caused by metabolic changes, prion disease, inflammatory disorders, neoplasm, infection of the brain and toxins. All of these will have unique profiles.

Chapter 3

DEMENTIA AND LOSS

Spend a few moments to think about the things in your life that are the most important to you. Not food, water or air, but the other things that are important which make you feel good or improve your quality of life.

> What is important to you?
> 1.
> 2.
> 3.

The specific things listed will be different for each of us but there are common themes for all of us. Family and friends are often listed as the most important, and pets, job, hobbies and home are also frequently included.

What if you had to give up one of the three things on your list? Think about it for a moment.

Which one would you choose? How easy is it to choose?

For the thing you have chosen, think about what it would it be like if you were never able to see this person, have this thing or do this activity again? How would this change your life?

Most of us take for granted the people and the things we have in our life and don't often consider what would happen if we had to give them up.

The things that are important to you – your family, job, home, leisure activities and so on – are all part of who you are.

Let's suppose one of the things that was important to you was going for a walk with your friend. What if you had an injury which meant that you could no longer walk long distances so you had to stop doing this? What would you do? You may be able to find another type of exercise or activity you enjoy and you could find other things to do with your friend. Hobbies are important, as they can improve the quality of our life, give us purposeful activity and increase social engagement.

What if your injury meant that you could no longer do your job and you had to give it up? Your job may be important to you for many reasons – it gives you a role and purpose, something to get up for in the morning and you enjoy it. We also usually need the money at the end of the month to pay our bills. You could plan and problem solve, try to get a new job and reduce your spending. What if you couldn't get another job and not working meant that you were no longer able to pay your rent or mortgage and had to move home? Moving home is one of the most stressful life events and is likely to be more so if it was not a choice you made. It may be harder to see family and friends following the move. What do you have left? How would this impact on the quality of your life? What would it be like if you gradually lost some of the things in your life that are important to you? It's difficult to think about this and it is certainly not something you would choose.

One of the experiences of dementia as it progresses is the loss of abilities, activities, people, and the things that are important to the person. We don't often put ourselves in the shoes of a person with dementia and think about the losses they experience and what it would feel like to live with these losses. If you engaged with the exercise above, it is likely that you had to think hard about what you would give up. You had a choice and it was just an exercise. A person living with dementia has no choice about the many losses they experience. People with dementia don't choose what they lose or the order in which they experience the loss. How we engage and support the person can contribute to their experience of loss or help them to adjust and develop ways to do things differently to cope with the loss.

Below are some of the losses which are associated with dementia.

LOSS OF MEMORY

We are all aware that dementia affects a person's memory but have you ever stopped to think about what that would feel like for the person?

Have you ever walked into a room and forgotten what you have gone in for? How does this make you feel? You may laugh to yourself and tell yourself that you need to slow down and pay more attention. You may feel annoyed with yourself or frustrated. What do you do? You stand in the room and think, mentally retrace your steps, trying to logically work out what it is you are looking for. You look for clues. What was I just doing? Where am I going? Sometimes you have to go back to where you started to remind you of what it was. Sometimes you can't recall and it's some time later before you remember and by this time it can be too late.

This happens to most of us occasionally. It happens to us usually when we are in a rush or not paying enough attention to what we are doing. As we get older it happens more often, but if a person has dementia, this can happen regularly. As these minor frustrations build up they can have a very negative impact on how the person feels. They may feel frustrated, angry with themselves, foolish or stupid, asking themselves, "why can't I remember such a small thing?" What impact would this have on self-esteem or sense of self?

Have you ever been lost in an unfamiliar place? I recall being lost in a country where I felt very unsafe and didn't speak the language. I had accidentally stepped off the main path. I had a map but I was frightened to take out the map because I didn't want to draw attention to myself. I didn't want to ask for directions as I was concerned that I may ask the wrong person who could take advantage of my vulnerability. Even without this fear, I didn't speak the language and would have been reliant on the likelihood of someone speaking English. Despite my anxiety, I was able to retrace my steps and find my way back to the main road. This was an experience I had over 20 years ago but I still remember the feelings of fear and anxiety. I had all my cognitive faculties and was able to plan and get out of the situation. What about a person with dementia who finds they are in a place they do not recognise? They may experience the same fear and anxiety. They may have impairment in language function and cannot ask for help. They may have problems in planning so cannot work out how to get to where they want to go. What if they are frightened to ask for help from strangers because they feel vulnerable? There is no difference between the fear and anxiety experienced by a person with dementia and my experience over 20 years ago. However, I was able to plan and retrace my steps and get back to a place where I felt safe. The person with dementia may be unable to do this. It's difficult to imagine what it would be like to have this experience frequently. Some people with dementia can regularly become lost in familiar environments. For them, the world can become a very frightening place where they feel vulnerable. How we engage with the person can either increase or decrease their fear and vulnerability.

What would it feel like if you couldn't remember what you had been doing the day before or earlier in the day? What if it was a wedding of a close friend, your child or grandchild? When you create a memory of an event you can look back on the event at a later time and smile when you think about it – it's a bit like reliving it. If you had no memory of that event, the inability to bring the event back into your mind would be a significant loss.

If you can't remember what happened, you may worry that you have said or done something wrong or upset someone. Or what if you did not recall what was going to happen later in the day? You may feel frightened and anxious and have a sense of uncertainty. You might seek assurance from others. You might ask family or friends what happened earlier or what is going to happen later. You may not ask, you may just feel stupid that you don't remember. When a person with dementia asks us about what has happened earlier or what is going to happen later, it is likely that they are trying to make sense of their day, reduce uncertainty and feel secure.

Think about when you are going somewhere new that you haven't been before and you don't quite know what to expect. You don't know who is going to be there or what you or they will be doing. You might possibly feel anxious. What if you had this experience all the time? The anxiety could be exhausting. How we interact with the person with dementia can reduce their anxiety and help them to feel safe.

What if you asked someone a question and they told you that they had answered that question 20 times already that day? How would this make you feel? It would most likely have an impact on your self-esteem, you may feel stupid, useless. We have all had experiences when we have forgotten something important, perhaps the birthday of a close friend. You may feel guilty or embarrassed. For most of us this is not a daily occurrence. For a person living with dementia, this happens every day and is likely to have a very negative impact on their mood and self-esteem. If we draw it to their attention, this is likely to make them feel worse.

LOSS OF ROLE

We all have many roles in our life; daughter/son, wife/husband, father/mother, brother/sister, employer/employee, friend, team player and many more. Our roles contribute to our sense of who we are, our purpose in life and our self-esteem.

Being a parent means different things to different people but it means something. You may be a parent who enjoys being part of your children's lives, offering love and support and helping with grandchildren. What if the dementia means that you can no longer be the parent you want to be? You're still the mother or father but your role has changed. The children and grandchildren that you once cared for are now helping to care for you.

What happens to your role as a husband or wife as dementia progresses? Throughout their marriage, a couple generally develop their roles within the family, some responsibilities are shared and some tend to be the responsibility of the husband or wife. There is shared decision making and problem solving, intimacy and trust in the relationship. The relationship changes with dementia and some of the roles within the marriage that the person with dementia generally completed are now completed by someone else. There is a loss of the traditional role of the husband or wife in the marriage. A new relationship develops but there is still a loss of what was normal. The relationship moves from partnership to being cared for. This is an unplanned change in role that can be very difficult to adjust to.

If a person living with dementia is still working, as the dementia progresses, they may have to make changes to how they do their job and eventually stop working. A person with dementia who is not in paid employment may still have many roles and responsibilities within and outside their home. If your role was to do the shopping, cooking, cleaning or DIY within the home and you were no longer able to independently do this, what is your role within the home now?

We all like to go on holiday to get away from everyday chores and relax. After two or three weeks on holiday we are usually glad to get back to our normal routine.

We want something to do. What would it be like to be on a permanent holiday from everyday chores but in a place you didn't choose where you have little to occupy you? What would it feel like to be permanently redundant? How would you spend your time? If you had dementia, would you still be able to spend your time doing these things? How would you feel? Would you be bored?

Having something to do is important to all of us. We all need to feel that we have a purpose. If we have no purpose, what's the point in getting out of bed? If you have nothing to do and there are no demands on your time, days would be long. Our roles, responsibilities and activities, in part, define who we are. If we have no role, then who are we? There is a risk that a person living with dementia could lose all of the roles and responsibilities that are important to them. If we are aware of this, however, we can stop it from happening.

LOSS OF SOCIAL CONTACT

Much of our social contact with other people involves us using language to communicate. If someone is talking to you and you don't understand, how does it make you feel? Have you ever been in a country where you don't speak the language? If someone starts talking to you and you don't understand what they are saying, you may feel embarrassed, frustrated or helpless and eventually you may give up trying to understand. It's more difficult to engage in social contact with people if you are unable to communicate with them using language; you have to be very creative to understand and be understood by others.

The person with dementia may find it more difficult to keep track of the conversation in a social setting. They may mishear or misunderstand what has been said and respond in a way that doesn't seem to fit with the conversation. The person may become aware that they have said the wrong thing because of the expression on other people's faces. If they have insight and are aware of their reduced ability to communicate, it can cause embarrassment and they may start to withdraw from social interaction.

Friends sometimes feel embarrassed or unsure about how best to engage with the person. Their relationship has changed and the normal pattern or conversation and interaction may no longer be appropriate. What do we talk about? What are we supposed to do? This can make friends feel uncomfortable.

Sometime when we visit there can be a pressure to make the visit worthwhile. Many of us have memories of visiting someone in hospital. The visiting time is relatively short and we are aware that the person may not have had visitors that day. We feel a sense of pressure to be interesting for that time. The visiting time can seem long if we run out of conversation. We are pleased if another visitor arrives, as it takes the pressure off us to be entertaining. While the context is very different to visiting someone with dementia, there are similarities if we don't know what to do, what to say or how to communicate.

It can be easier not to visit. We all have busy lives and we might find that we are tied up and less able to visit. This is not necessarily a conscious decision but we may find other things which need to be done during a time when we would normally have visited. Some people may believe that their visit is of no benefit to the person and they will not recall the visit.

Throughout our day, we have many opportunities to engage in social interaction, when working, out and about, shopping, participating in a hobby or attending church. Many people with dementia lose access to these activities, which can result in an increasing loss of social contact.

The person with dementia may not engage in the same way but they can still enjoy the experience of social interaction. Our sense of wellbeing is made up of all the experiences we have across the day. It's not just one experience that matters but all of them together. If the person with dementia has multiple positive experiences throughout the day, this will have a positive impact on their wellbeing even if they don't recall the specific events. The positive emotion experienced can continue to have a very positive impact even after the visit.

LOSS OF RELATIONSHIP

When a person is diagnosed with dementia this impacts on the person, their family and friends.

Social contact and relationships with other people are important to us. Relationships change as dementia progresses, and new ways of making connections need to be found. This is not always easy and there can be significant stress around the transition as relationships adapt to the changes that come with dementia. These adaptations are not always easy to make and relationships can be lost along the way.

As the person with dementia becomes less able to independently visit friends they are more dependent on other people visiting them to maintain the relationship. Other people may not always think about visiting or have time to visit. As discussed above, family and work commitments get in the way. The ability to communicate may be reduced and behaviour or personality may have changed. Friends and family can find visiting more challenging. The person may not recognise you. Friends may feel uncomfortable visiting or they may feel that their visit is not wanted. Dementia may mean that there is a change in the relationship but this does not mean that the relationship is less valuable. By continuing to engage with and visit them, you are helping to prevent another loss of something very important.

Family can have a similar experience. It was discussed above how husband and wife relationships can move from a partnership to a carer role. This can impact on the relationship and there can be a loss of partnership and intimacy. It can also be difficult for families to negotiate the changes in communication, personality and behaviour that may come with dementia. It can be difficult to visit your mother or father when they no longer behave in the way that they did before. The relationship has changed, something is lost, the love is still there but something about the relationship is very different. Finding new ways to maintain the relationship bonds is important for both the person with dementia and their family. They are all experiencing the loss.

It can be distressing to see someone you love change and experience the losses associated with dementia. The distress experienced when we visit someone we love and see how they have changed can make it difficult to visit. We may want to remember the person as they were before the dementia. At other times, the person can become distressed when the visit is ending and you are leaving. The distress is experienced by both parties and can lead us to question whether we are in fact making things worse by visiting.

When someone moves into a care home, friends and families may visit very regularly at the start but as time goes on they find that they are less able to visit as often as they would like to or the person with dementia would like them to. It can be an emotional experience, particularly if you would prefer to have the person at home with you but you are unable to provide the care they need. There are many emotions experienced, and this can be worse if the person is not settled in their new home. This separation, forced by circumstances, can place a significant strain on the relationship.

What if family and friends live far away and the person is no longer able to use the phone, read or write letters, texts or emails? Having dementia doesn't change the importance of the relationship. The person with dementia can still miss someone even if they cannot tell us this. We may be able to help to maintain these relationships by looking and talking about photographs, reminiscing about the person and talking about what they are doing now. This may be helpful for some people, depending on the stage of their dementia.

Current relationships with friends, family and work colleagues are based on your recollection of the person and previous encounters with them. What if you couldn't recognise the person or remember what your relationship was? You may miss that person even if they are standing in front of you because you don't recognise who they are. If this happens it would be important to find ways to maintain the relationship. Trying to tell the person who you are may add to their distress if they do not recognise you. You may be able to use old photographs of a time where they do recognise who you are to engage with them. This may be a way of bringing a younger version of you into their mind, even if they don't recognise who you are now.

The new relationships we build with friends, family, neighbours, carers and work colleagues are based on our recollection of previous encounters we have with these people. We develop relationships with people because we remember previous occasions when we met them, what we did, how they behaved and interacted with us and whether we had a good time together. We develop good friendships because we have positive shared experiences and our memory for these shared experiences helps us to build friendship bonds. With work colleagues, our memory of previous encounters also shapes these relationships. Can we trust that person? Do they do a good job? Do they "have my back"? When a person has dementia, how can we help them to build new relationships even if they cannot remember their previous encounters with people? It may be more about the relationship in the moment. If we can make the experience a positive one, then we have a safe relationship in that moment. This can be particularly important for people who move into a care home or have carers coming into their home whom they do not know.

We have all had the experience of meeting someone and feeling that this is a person I could get on with or this is a person I would not choose to spend a lot of time with. Two people may do or say the same thing but there is something that is different. You can't quite put your finger on it but it's different. It could be a lot of things, their tone of voice, their body language, and the way they look at you. These things and many more add up to enable us to form a positive or negative impression of someone. The same is true with a person with dementia. The way you engage with them will be what determines their impression of you. The feeling of being respected and safe is very important. That feeling of safety and security from the interaction can linger through the day.

Maintaining a connection may be easier if we don't rely solely on language. Finding an activity to engage in with the person with dementia can help to maintain the connection or build a new relationship. When we spend time with a friend or family member with dementia, if we have an activity we can do together it makes the time more meaningful. Similarly for care staff, engaging in an activity with a person with dementia helps to build and maintain relationships.

LOSS OF HOME

What does home mean? What makes a home feel like a home? Home is not the bricks and mortar, it's the people and the memories associated with the things inside that make it home. Our family, neighbours, bed, chair, cup and many more things. Home is associated with a feeling of safety and security.

What if you no longer recognised your home? As dementia progresses the person may ask to go home, even if they are in their own home. They may no longer recognise the people or things around them as familiar. Sometimes family will believe that they want to go to a place where they lived in the past. Family may even bring the person back to a former dwelling to help to reduce distress. This generally does not work because usually it is not what the person is looking for. When they are looking for home they are most likely looking for the feelings that home brings, feelings of comfort, safety and security. When this happens, we need to find ways to help the person to feel more comfortable, safe and secure. Sometimes this can be with positive interaction, photographs, music and activity. The way we talk to and engage with the person can help them to feel safe.

What if the person has to move home, move into supported accommodation or a care home? They may lose many of the things that represent home, the things which trigger memories of their past and help them to feel comfortable, safe and secure.

What would it be like to move from your home into a care home? For some people with dementia, this is something they chose, for others it isn't their choice. Whether it was something chosen by the person or not, moving home is a very stressful life event. Moving to a new environment when you have dementia can be an even more stressful experience.

As discussed above, if we form positive relationships with people through our recollections of previous positive encounters with them, how do people with dementia do this when they move into a care home? They wake up in the morning and people whom they don't know come into their room to offer support. They go into a communal dining room for breakfast with other people they don't know. Throughout the day, people whom they don't know come and go. If they can't remember that they are in a care home and who these people are, how do they know if they are safe? Who they can trust? Who is friendly and who is not?

The person with dementia may not know who the staff are. Care staff may need to introduce themselves on every occasion that they meet the person. "Hello, I'm Sally, a care worker." If you take your time and have a friendly expression this can help the person with dementia to feel that you are safe and they don't need to be anxious. When you leave, they may have no recollection of the experience but they will remember how you made them feel. Did you make them feel respected, cared for and safe? If you did, the more often you engage with the person the less likely they are to feel anxious when you offer support. While they may not remember individual encounters, they will have the feeling that this is a safe place. If the person feels safe, the interaction will be better and it will be a good experience for both of you.

We often don't think about whether the person chose to move to a care home or indeed chose to live in the specific care home they now live in. We take it for granted that they just live there. We fail to acknowledge the significant losses they have experienced on their journey from their own home to the care home and how that may make them feel.

What if you had limited or no choice about where you lived or whom you lived with? People living with dementia in care homes have no choice about the other residents who live there. They may get on with some of the residents or they may have nothing in common with any of them. If their memory is poor, they may not recall that they are in a care home and who these other people are.

Have you ever been on holiday and woken up, forgotten you were on holiday and wondered where you are? You probably remember very quickly. But what if you have dementia and wake up in your room in a care home where the surroundings are not familiar? The walls are a different colour, the furniture is different. There are some things that seem familiar but it's just not right. Then someone you do not know comes into your room. How would you feel? Would you feel scared? How would you react? This happens to people living with dementia every day.

What about the furniture, the decor, the bed? If you have been away from home you always look forward to getting home and getting into your own bed for a good night's sleep.

Eating in a communal dining room every day is not what most of us call normal life. This may happen when we go on holiday or go out for a meal, but not every day. Even when we do eat out, we normally sit with family or friends. How often do we sit at a table with other people whom we do not know well? They may or may not have language skills to engage in conversation with us. What is going on? Where am I? Why am I here? When can I go home? I don't like the food. I don't like these people at my table.

What would you do? Get up and leave. When a person in a care home gets up to leave the table what happens? Staff usually ask them to sit down again to eat their meal. Why is she asking me to sit down? I want to go home. If the person refuses to sit down, what happens?

You are sitting in a lounge with other people you do not know. They may behave in ways that are unpredictable. Some of them walk around, some of them shout, some are sleeping. What is going on? Where are my family and friends? Where is the toilet? I want to make myself a cup of tea. I want a snack. I want to go out for a walk. I want to do my washing. I want fish and chips from the local chip shop for tea.

When we are aware of the possible feelings of being unsafe and the multiple losses associated with moving into a care home, we are more able to see life from the perspective of the person. When we do this, we improve the quality of our interaction with them and the quality of their life.

LOSS OF FAMILIAR ROUTINES

Most of us are creatures of habit. We sometimes do things spontaneously but generally we are fairly predictable. We usually get up around the same time and eat our meals around the same time each day. Even with the foods we eat we tend to have the same breakfast most mornings and have a relatively small range of foods that we eat for lunch and dinner. We shop in the same supermarket each week and have favourite brands of food that we buy. When you think about most of the activities you do throughout the week, you probably do most of them at set times on set days along with the same group of people.

A set routine gives us predictability and security; we know where we are and what we're doing. There are occasions when we break from routine, either planned or unplanned, but largely there are fixed patterns in our behaviour. Dementia can throw all of this into a spin as the person may no longer be able to do some of the things they did before. The routine can be lost and with this loss can come feelings of uncertainty and insecurity. To help with this we need to support the person to develop a new routine, one that is predictable and can help them to feel more secure. It is important to help the person to do things differently, or at a different time, or find an alternative activity to build into a routine.

A person who has moved house or moved into a care home will experience a significant change in routine. They will need support to adjust and develop a new routine in this new environment.

LOSS OF INDEPENDENCE

We all enjoy our independence and making our own decisions. We don't like to be dependent on other people. What would it be like if you were no longer free to do what you wanted when you wanted? What if you needed support from others to do some or all of your activities of daily living?

It's great when people do something for us sometimes, such as making us a cup of tea or cooking dinner. What would it be like if you depended on someone to make you a cup of tea or make your dinner every time? This would be a very different experience. Other people don't always do things exactly as we would choose to do them or at a time when we want to do them. What if you needed support to bathe and dress? This can be particularly difficult for some people who are very private. It can be a very uncomfortable experience for the person to receive support from family or paid carers with intimate tasks of personal care such as using the toilet, bathing and dressing. For a person who has always been independent, the reduced ability to meet every day needs can be very difficult to adjust to. People can experience a range of emotions from frustration, anger and embarrassment to helplessness. There can be a sense of loss of control over your own life.

LOSS OF ACTIVITY

A person may be less able to engage in the activities they previously enjoyed because of a change in their ability to do these activities. Or they may no longer be able to travel to activities independently so cannot access activities. For example, a person may have regularly attended their church or social group but may be unable to do this independently anymore.

All of the roles and social interaction discussed above are activities. Loss of these things adds up to a loss of purposeful activity.

If we think about the perspective of the person with dementia and consider the potential losses they experience, we can change how we engage with them. By making very simple changes to what we do we can significantly improve the experience the person has as they navigate through their day and help them to live well, despite the losses that come with dementia.

Chapter 4

DEMENTIA AND SENSE OF SELF

Our sense of self is our personal identity, who we are, and it is made up of many things:

- Family relationships – such as husband/wife; brother/sister; son/daughter; mother/father.
- Other relationships – such as friend, work colleague.
- Occupation – what we do for a living.
- Roles – such as problem solver, baby sitter, volunteer.
- Hobbies.
- Associations – teams we support, groups and societies we are members of.
- Strengths and weaknesses – such as smart, funny, impatient.
- Qualities – such as good friend, reliable, determined, hardworking.
- Spirituality – beliefs or religion.

Our sense of self is connected to our ability to make a contribution in our various relationships, roles and everyday activities. What happens to their sense of self when a person starts to lose their ability to make the same contribution to these things?

How does dementia impact on sense of self?

Changes to sense of self depend on the stage of dementia and the support available to help the person to adjust and compensate for changes in their ability.

It is easy to see how dementia has the potential to impact on sense of self. The loss in roles and relationships discussed in Chapter 3 are the very things that make up our sense of self. Completing household tasks and engaging in hobbies may be difficult, there may be a shift from helper to helpee and relationships with friends and family can change.

Changes in abilities and relationships don't necessarily have to lead to a negative change in sense of self. Our sense of self also depends on our experiences as we interact with the world and other people. Our experience of interacting with others and how they treat us influences what we believe about ourselves. If someone is polite and respectful, we feel valued as a person. If someone is rude, disrespectful or dismissive, it can make us feel devalued as a person.

There are many ways in which how we behave can determine how another person with or without dementia feels. Throughout the day there are many opportunities to treat other people in such a way that they experience a sense of achievement and feel valued as a person with something to contribute. By engaging with them in a different way, we can cause them to experience a sense of failure and feel that they have nothing to offer. It doesn't have to be anything special. Just taking the time to say "Hello" to someone can be enough to make them feel valued.

What happens when we fail?

Think about the last time you were trying to do something and couldn't do it. One example that comes to mind is reversing a car into a small parking space. Many drivers find this difficult. What if you had a few attempts and couldn't get in? How would this make you feel? You might feel like a failure. You might feel embarrassed, particularly if there was someone else in the car with you, other people watching or a queue of traffic waiting behind you. What would you do? You might keep trying until you get into the space or, depending on the circumstances, you may just give up and drive off.

People with dementia have this type of experience every day. Not with parking a car, but with things that they could normally have done very easily and can no longer do without many attempts and frequent failures. Their experience of frustration and failure is no different from our experience if we are unable to reverse into a parking space. The difference is that we can choose not to use the small space and find a different parking space. A person with dementia experiences challenges multiple times throughout every day with many of their essential activities of daily living. These challenges can start at the beginning of each day when they get up and try to get dressed. The challenges continue throughout the day until they are in bed at night. Even when they are in bed at night dementia can impact on their sleep.

Think about getting dressed in the morning. You may pay attention to choosing what to wear but pay little attention to the rest of it. Taking off your night clothes and putting on day clothes you do almost automatically without thinking about it. Getting dressed is a fairly complex task, but because you have been doing it for years it appears to be simple. For a person with dementia this can be difficult. Getting dressed requires a number of cognitive processes, including memory, planning, organising and sequencing. Below are just some of the steps involved:

- Be aware that it is day time.
- Remember that there are different clothes for day and night.
- Make a decision to change out of your night clothes.
- Consider the weather and what you will be doing that day.
- Make a decision about what clothing to wear, weighing up all the necessary information.
- Remember where your clothes are kept – what items are kept in the wardrobe, chest of drawers and so on.
- Find all the clothes you need.
- Remove your night clothing.
- Put your new clothes on in the correct order and the right way round.

When you realise how complex this task is and how many steps and processes are involved, it is easy to see how a person with dementia may have difficulty with one or more of the steps. If you fail at the beginning of the day and throughout the day, how will this make you feel? By offering appropriate support, but not taking over, we can turn this potential failure into a success. What step or steps is the person finding difficult because of their dementia? Can we offer support in a respectful way with these steps to enable them to complete the other steps independently?

Have you ever been doing something and someone else took over because you "weren't doing it properly" or you "weren't doing it fast enough"? What about the reverse parking example. What if you had someone in the car with you telling you to hurry up because there was a queue of traffic behind you? Would this have helped your parking? No, it would be unlikely to help you, it would be more likely to make you feel anxious. Your anxiety may, in turn, make it less likely that you would successfully park the car. What if your passenger told you to get out of the car and they would park. Part of you may feel relieved but another part of you would feel that you had failed. If they parked the car with relative ease this would add to your feelings of inadequacy and incompetence.

When people with dementia are no longer able to complete all their activities of daily living and we remind them that they are not doing it properly or fast enough, how will they feel? How might they feel if we take over and do it for them? They will have the same feelings of inadequacy and incompetence as we have when someone else has to park the car for us. In the dressing example, if the person with dementia no longer knows the order in which to put their clothes on, if we lay the clothes out for them, they may be able to get dressed independently, even if it takes longer. Supporting someone to be as independent as possible is a very different experience for that person than taking over and doing it for them.

We can recover from the car parking experience if we have opportunities for success in other things we do. We have all had experiences of failure but when these failures are infrequent we can "put it down to experience", "learn from it" and "move on" – for example, "I may not be able to reverse park but I can…" How would it feel if you had multiple failures in your day and few opportunities for success? Your concept of self is likely to be as a failure or someone who is incompetent or useless. We need to ensure that people living with dementia have experiences where they can successfully complete tasks

What happens when we succeed?

Think about a time when you did something well. It doesn't have to be anything special. Perhaps a time when you had invited friends or relatives for dinner. You may have gone to a lot of trouble to cook the meal. Beforehand you may have worried that it would all go well. On the day, the food tasted great and everyone had a good time. How did you feel? Most likely you felt really good, a sense of achievement.

Positive feedback is very rewarding. How do you feel when someone says, "Thanks, that was really helpful" or "You're doing a great job"? Your sense of self is likely to be that you are appreciated, a person who has something worthwhile to contribute. When someone compliments you on what you have done you usually feel good. The acknowledgement of a job well done increases your self-esteem.

How do you feel when you have been doing something that you found really difficult and finished it? You may feel a sense of achievement and satisfaction. You usually feel good about yourself, which also has a positive impact on your self-esteem.

Supporting a person with dementia to access and engage in purposeful meaningful activity will ensure that they have the opportunity to experience purpose, success and a sense of achievement. This will have a positive impact on their self-esteem and quality of life. Activities need to be appropriate for the person's level of ability. If we evaluate a person's achievements based on their ability before dementia, the person will fall short. It is important to have an understanding of what their level of ability is and support them to complete tasks and activities at this level. It may be necessary to be creative in identifying a range of meaningful activities and tasks in which the person has the opportunity to experience success and a sense of having achieved something and made a contribution.

Our sense of self also contributes to our motivation. If we believe we are good at something, we will be motivated to do it. If we believe we are not good at something, we will be less motivated to do it. For a person with dementia who may experience challenges completing many activities of daily living, it is easy to see how they begin to lose motivation, for example, "I can't do it, what's the point in trying." If we offer appropriate support to maintain as much independence as possible and facilitate success, we will increase motivation. We can do this by supporting any areas of weakness, slowing the pace at which a task is completed, breaking the task into steps and taking one step at a time. For some types of dementia, the reduced motivation is a direct consequence of the area of the brain that is damaged rather than the psychological experience of multiple failures. Even if this is the case, increasing independence and the opportunity for success will still have a positive impact on the experience of the person.

We can change how the person experiences the world by supporting them to experience success, ensuring that they feel they have something to offer and have a purpose each day. We don't have to do anything difficult to achieve this. If we are respectful and provide opportunities for them to engage with other people and have something to do this will have a positive impact on their self-esteem and sense of self.

Chapter 5

UNDERSTANDING BEHAVIOUR

Why do we behave the way we do? That's a difficult question to answer because the answer depends on what the behaviour is and a range of different factors.

SALLY'S STORY

Sally gets up at 7am, takes a shower and gets dressed. She wakes her two children to get up for school. She goes downstairs and her husband is preparing breakfast – two pieces of wholemeal bread, lightly toasted with a little butter and orange marmalade. She makes a cup of tea, not too strong, with semi-skimmed milk. Sally organises the cereal for their children and helps them to get organised for school. She leaves the house at 8.15am, drops her children at school and drives to work. She finishes work at 4pm, picks the children up from their after-school club and helps them with their homework. She prepares dinner, stew on a Tuesday. Later she gets the children organised for bed and watches her favourite TV programme and is in bed by 11pm.

There is nothing particularly unusual about Sally's day. What if you were told that at 7.15am Sally got up from her chair in the kitchen and left the house? Why do you think she did that? How could you possibly know? You don't have enough information about Sally to know why she behaved in the way she did. You could guess that she needed something from the shop or that she had arranged to meet a friend. Without more information about Sally, you wouldn't know.

SUSAN'S STORY

Susan gets up at 7.30am, washes her face, gets dressed and puts her make-up on. She drinks a glass of orange juice and eats a bowl of cereal while watching breakfast TV. She leaves the house at 8.15am and drives to work. She finishes work at 5pm, goes to the gym and gets home around 7pm. She prepares dinner, pasta. She listens to some music while reading a book and is in bed by 11pm.

Again, there is nothing particularly unusual about Susan's day. What if you were told that at 7.15am Susan got up off her chair in the kitchen and left the house. Why do you think she did that? Do you think it was for the same reason that Sally left her home at 7.15am? How could you possibly know?

We have two people engaging in the same behaviour but we do not know why. What if you were told that Sally shouted at her daughter at 5pm on Tuesday? What would you think about Sally? Is she impatient? Is she a bad mother for not being able to control her temper? You might want to know how often she shouts at her daughter. Is it something that happens regularly or infrequently? You would want to know what her daughter was doing before Sally shouted at her that may have caused Sally to shout. If you knew that Sally rarely shouted at her daughter or frequently shouted at her daughter, this would have an impact on what you think about Sally. What if her daughter was about to touch a hot pan on the stove? You might conclude that her shouting was an appropriate response to try to protect her daughter from harm. What if her daughter had refused to do her homework, had been fighting with her brother and had just eaten a packet of sweets that Sally had asked her to save until after dinner? You may feel that shouting was not an appropriate response but you may also understand why she shouted. What if Sally was just recovering from an illness, was tired or had a headache. You may feel that it was unfair to shout at her daughter but she lost her patience because of her illness. What this highlights is that the "shouting" behaviour is the same but there are a number of potential explanations for this behaviour. There are also a number of factors which contribute to the behaviour: Sally's personality, how she is feeling, and her daughter's behaviour are only a few of the possible factors.

This gives a flavour on how complex our behaviour really is. There is never just one factor that determines what we do or why we behave in the way we do.

JOHN'S STORY

John is a 79-year-old man sitting in a chair in the lounge of a care home waving his walking stick in the air, shouting, but it is not clear what he is saying. Why is he doing this? What does he want? Is he aggressive? Are staff or the other residents around him at risk of harm?

John was diagnosed with Alzheimer's disease two years ago and has been living in the care home for six months. John's mobility is poor and he uses a stick to support him when walking but also needs the assistance of one other person. It's 10am and John had porridge and a cup of tea for breakfast. After breakfast, staff supported John to sit in the lounge. The staff are in the middle of their medication round, which is a very busy time for them. Two members of staff are at the medication trolley near the lounge door sorting out the medication for residents.

John calls out, "nurse!" Because of his dementia, his language is not clear so it doesn't sound like "nurse" to others. There is a TV on in the room and the staff don't hear John. He calls out again, louder this time, "nurse!", but the staff still don't hear. He raises his voice again but is not heard above the noise of the TV. He lifts his stick to wave it to attract their attention.

John is generally quite a placid man. He gets frustrated with himself at times as he is more dependent on other people. He always enjoyed being active but his mobility has slowed him down. He thinks to himself, "What has life come to, I can't even get to the toilet on my own." He is continent but his reduced mobility means that he needs support from one member of staff to get from the lounge to the bathroom. His speech is impaired so he finds it difficult to tell people what he wants. He can understand what other people are saying if they speak slowly and clearly.

By the time the nurse realises that John is trying to attract her attention, what she sees is John raising his stick and almost hitting another resident with it. She has no knowledge that John had been trying to attract her attention for the past few minutes. The nurse rushes over and tells John to put his stick down as he might hit the other resident sitting beside him. To the staff member, this is a physically aggressive act. But is it? It wasn't John's intention to be aggressive, he was trying to attract the nurse's attention but could not be heard, so in his opinion at the time, waving his stick to attract attention was his best option. He had no intention of trying to hurt anyone and did not think that his stick could have potentially hurt another resident. He is confused by the nurse's alarmed expression, he just needs the toilet.

John has prostrate problems and urinary urgency. By the time the nurse reached John he had been incontinent because he was unable to control his bladder during the delay. John is embarrassed by the incontinence and when the nurse supports him to change his clothing he appears to be cross with her. John's behaviour is interpreted as physical aggression (shaking his stick at another resident), verbal aggression (being cross with staff when they are trying to help him) and resisting support with personal care (John was embarrassed when staff had to support him to change his clothes and resisted staff attempts to remove his trousers). Staff are trying to be supportive, they haven't done anything wrong, and cannot understand why he is so cross with them. John is not cross with them, he is frustrated with his reduced mobility and his problems with communication and is embarrassed by his incontinence which is a direct result of his prostrate difficulties and his inability to attract attention when he needs it.

The staff didn't realise John had been trying to attract their attention to go to the toilet. Because of his communication difficulties and his embarrassment he cannot tell them that he had been trying to call them. If someone is cross with us when we are only trying to help them, this can change how we respond to them. We may be less friendly. Staff may become a bit more wary of John as they don't want to get hit with his stick if "he decides to become aggressive again". The incontinence has had a significant impact on John and he is more withdrawn and engages less with staff and other residents. In this case, it's not that anyone has done anything wrong. An unfortunate set of circumstances arose which caused distress for John, and the care staff may now feel that he is ungrateful and unappreciative of the support that they are offering. His behaviour may be misinterpreted as "aggression" as a consequence of his dementia. They have not seen the context which would help them to understand his behaviour.

Two days later a similar thing happens. This time the nurse does hear him after his second attempt to call out to attract her attention. She is in the middle of sorting out the medication for a resident and says, "I will be with you in a minute John." Five minutes pass and she is still busy. John's urgency to use the toilet increases and he shouts again and raises his stick. By the time the nurse reaches him he has been incontinent again. He is embarrassed, ashamed, cross with himself because he is dependent on others to use the toilet.

Staff have the impression that this is a deterioration in his dementia. He is becoming physically aggressive and incontinent. It is suggested that he wear pads to manage his incontinence. This has a further negative impact on John's self-esteem and he resists attempts from staff to support him to use an incontinence pad. "I don't need a nappy, nappies are for babies. I can go to the toilet on my own if someone can help me to walk there."

This example shows how easy it is to misinterpret the behaviour and intentions of others and the impact this can then have on how we interact with them and treat them. How do we ever really know why someone behaves in a certain way? If I get up from my chair, it's not just a random act, it has a purpose. I may want to make a cup of tea, use the bathroom or I may just want a change of scenery. The only way to really know why I got up from my chair is to ask me. People with dementia are no different from all of us. Their behaviour also has a purpose. They may not have the language skills to tell you why they are behaving in a certain way or what it is that they want. If a person living with dementia cannot use language to tell us what they need, we need to find the clues to help us to understand what they need.

Behaviour is a form of communication. Interpreting the communication requires "listening" to the behaviours.

When someone with dementia has been sitting in the same chair for a while, they may also want to get up to walk around, just like anyone else may want to do. If this happens in a care home, the behaviour can sometimes be described as "wandering" or "pacing". Is this really wandering or is it simply going for a walk and getting a change of scenery? There may be many reasons why someone will walk around their home. They may be looking for a particular object, looking for the toilet or going to look for something to eat. We may call this wandering but we don't really know why the person is walking. We rarely go wandering, we are usually walking with some purpose, to get a change of scenery, fresh air, to go to a shop, to get something from another room.

CLEAR Dementia Care© (Duffy 2016; Duffy and Richardson 2018) was developed to help carers understand behaviour in people living with dementia. It provides simple tools to help carers see when specific behaviours happen, as this is extremely important when trying to understand the behaviour (see Chapter 6). CLEAR Dementia Care© also helps carers to see that there are a number of factors or domains which contribute to a person's behaviour. These domains are explained in greater detail in Chapter 8. When we consider all the factors that may contribute to a behaviour we have a greater understanding of why the behaviour is happening and what the person needs.

If we can see the whole person in the context of the life they are living, we will be better able to understand their behaviour. A person may appear to be restless, not wanting to sit down and wishing to frequently walk around. When we offer support, the person may resist our help and may appear to hit out, verbally or physically. This behaviour is often a sign of the stress and distress the person experiences as they try to meet their needs, tell others what they need, understand what is happening around them or cope with the daily challenges of living with their condition. If we are able to understand their needs, support them to meet these needs and help them to understand what is happening around them, we will reduce the distress that is associated with these behaviours.

We all develop unique ways of understanding, interacting and coping with daily life. What do you do if you have had a stressful day at home or at work? You may read, watch television, get some exercise, phone a friend or have a drink. What does a person with dementia do if they are having a bad day? Most likely they will want to do what they have always done. What if this was phoning a friend? They may no longer have access to a phone, be able to use the phone or be unable to explain how they are feeling or why they are feeling this way. What if they would normally have gone for a walk? If they try to leave their home or a care home, what will happen? Most likely someone will try to stop them or in some cases they will be unable to leave as the door may be locked for safety. How will that make the person feel? What impact will that have on their stress? It is likely to increase their distress.

People with dementia have bad days too, just like the rest of us. When this happens, they will need to have things to do or people to support them. How can we help people with dementia to find ways to cope with the stresses of everyday life? The answer is we try to better understand what they want and find ways to help them to meet their needs.

People with dementia have the same needs as everyone else and continue to try to find ways to meet their needs. The way in which they interact and communicate their needs has changed, because of the impact dementia has had on their ability to think and express themselves using language. To find out what their needs are at a particular time and help them help to meet their needs we need to see the world from their perspective (Kitwood 1997).

IT'S ALL ABOUT PERSPECTIVE

Imagine you have been in work all day, it's the end of your shift, and you want to go home to your family. As you reach the door the boss calls you back and says you can't leave, you need to stay at least another hour as there is a crisis. The other staff go home, you have to watch them leave while you remain somewhere you don't really want to be. How do you feel? You may feel angry or frustrated. What do you do? If you have to stay, you may need to make plans. You may have arranged to meet friends after work. You could telephone and tell them you will be late. You may have children to collect from school so you will need to make alternative arrangements for them. What if there is no one else who can collect your children from school?

Do you stay in work? If you think your children will be standing at the school gates alone, are you happy to stay in work? Most likely not. You will attempt to leave to get your children. What if your boss tries to stop you? Will you be calm and comply with your boss's request and risk your children being unsafe? No, you will refuse to stay and if your boss persists you will no doubt become agitated and potentially aggressive if he or she continues to stop you from leaving. Your priority is to ensure that your children are safe.

What do you think that Carol, standing at the locked door in a care home is thinking and feeling when she tells staff that she has "to go home to the children"? There may be no children waiting for her at home but for her, the time she believes she is living in, there are real children at home. When Carol is prevented from leaving, her level of distress will escalate as she worries about the safety of her children. Asking her to come and sit down and have a cup of tea is unlikely to help. Would it help for you in this situation?

If we are prevented from leaving work, we can make arrangements to ensure our children are safe. If we have made plans to go for dinner we can contact friends to tell them we will be late. A person with dementia who believes they have to be somewhere else doesn't have the opportunity to do this. To support Carol, we need to look at her day, look for the patterns in her behaviour. When does she go to the door? If she was engaged in an activity, would she be less likely to go to the door? Is she missing her children? Would it help to look at pictures of her family and reminisce? Does she feel the need to care for someone? Would doll therapy be appropriate for Carol? There are many potential ways to reduce Carol's distress but first we need a greater understanding of when Carol becomes distressed and more information about Carol and her life. When we have a greater understanding of Carol, we can find ways to support her (see Chapters 6 and 8).

When a person with dementia is attempting to leave or engaging in another behaviour that we do not understand, the challenge for us is to try to understand their perspective. The person with dementia may not have the ability to see our perspective so they will not understand why we are asking them to do something that is inconsistent with their view of the situation. We have the ability to try to see their perspective. What are they are trying to do? Why are they trying to do this? Do they understand what is happening?

We interpret what people say and do according to a number of things which includes our past experiences, culture and values. This is also the case for dementia. How we understand dementia and behaviour in dementia depends on our understanding and beliefs about dementia. If we believe that people with dementia are unpredictable, they wander about and can be aggressive, then we will interpret their behaviour in terms of wandering and aggression. If we understand that a person with dementia is no different from us then we will interpret their behaviour differently. We can try to think, if I was in their shoes what would I do? The more we understand about the person with dementia, the easier it will be for us to see the world from their perspective. The domains of CLEAR Dementia Care© (Chapter 8) help us to do this.

We constantly try to make sense of the world, we make judgements and form opinions about every event and interaction. This sense-making is based on our previous experience which means that we see the world through coloured glasses and everyone has different glasses as they have had different experiences. What happens when a person has dementia? People with dementia continue to try to understand, react and respond to the world around them. The world they now live in can sometimes be a confusing, frightening and unfamiliar place that they have difficulty understanding.

For some people with dementia, their timeline might have shifted. When they interpret the world, it may be as a 40-year-old who is still working and has children at home, although in fact, they may be 82 years old and living in a care home. If as carers we can understand this then we can offer support to the 82-year-old without increasing distress.

Sometimes if we are in a situation that we are very close to or is causing us some emotional distress it is hard for us to know what is happening. The expression, "you can't see the wood for the trees" captures this. Stepping back from a situation often allows us to see the bigger picture. This can be the case if we are engaging with someone who appears to be aggressive. We may be frightened for ourselves or others, and emotions can be high. In an emotionally charged situation it is more difficult to accurately interpret and fully understand what is happening.

When we step back from a situation, we are better able to think about how others might see the situation differently. Seeing different perspectives helps to change our interpretation, reduce the emotion associated with the situation and helps us to be more understanding and empathic.

Imagine you are lying in bed at home feeling very cosy under the duvet. You hear a noise and a stranger walks into the room. How are you feeling? Most likely scared. Who is this person? How did they get in here? What do they want? Are they going to hurt me? They walk towards you and start speaking but you don't understand what they are saying. As they approach you are becoming more frightened. They continue talking and try to remove your duvet. You resist and try to defend yourself. They persist, another person enters the room and there are now two people trying to remove the duvet. You're terrified. You try to hit out to defend yourself. They are both talking to you but you don't understand what they are saying. They start to remove your clothing all the time talking to you but you have no idea what they are saying. "Why is this happening to me?" "What are they going to do to me?" You try to resist as much as possible but it is two against one. You are terrified, shouting out and trying to fight them off.

This is the experience of many people like Teresa living with dementia every day. A care worker, a stranger, comes into her room to support her to get dressed. Teresa, because of her dementia doesn't understand what is happening and believes she is being robbed and assaulted. She is terrified and starts to hit out at the stranger to defend herself. The care worker has come in, said good morning to Teresa and told Teresa who she is. Teresa doesn't understand because she has communication difficulties. The care worker has no idea that Teresa is frightened and doesn't understand why Teresa is trying to hit her; she hasn't done anything to harm Teresa. The care worker sees Teresa as a person who is physically aggressive because of her dementia. The care worker understandably finds it difficult to work with Teresa. The care worker may have become hurt as Teresa tries to resist her support and defend herself. Nobody wants to go to work to be hit by someone they are only trying to help. The care worker doesn't understand that Teresa is a scared and vulnerable lady who doesn't know that the care worker is safe and is only there to help her to get up. The care worker discusses this with her manager and it is agreed that two people are required to support Teresa in the morning. Now Teresa has two people who enter her room every morning. Teresa's family don't understand her aggression as she has always been a very mild-mannered lady. There is a risk that if Teresa's distress continues a decision will be made that she can no longer be supported with personal care in the morning.

Every person involved in a situation has their unique perspective of that situation. Neither Teresa nor the care worker has done anything wrong. It is likely that if any of us had their perspective and were not aware of the other person's perspective we would have done the same as they did. With a greater understanding of Teresa's perspective, the distress could have been avoided.

To understand behaviour, we need to take into consideration all the factors that may be contributing to the situation/behaviour and try to see the world from the perspective of the person with dementia (see Chapter 8). This requires looking beyond the label of dementia to find the person. The challenge is to find the clues and meet the person's needs.

Chapter 6

RECORDING BEHAVIOUR

Chapter 5 highlights that to understand behaviour we need some idea of when the behaviour occurs. To do this, CLEAR Dementia Care© uses Behaviour Record Charts (see Appendix 1), which were developed through experience of working in care homes with the Northern Health and Social Care Trust Dementia Home Support Team. People with dementia are referred to this specialist service when they present with behaviours that care staff find difficult to understand and the behaviour is causing distress for the person and the staff.

Prior to the development of CLEAR Dementia Care©, the team were using the Newcastle model working in care homes. The Newcastle model (James 2011) is a biopsychosocial model that promotes assessment and consideration of the range of factors which may be contributing to a particular behaviour. One of the tools used to help assess and understand behaviour is Antecedent Behaviour Consequence (ABC) charts. ABC charts require staff to record the *antecedent* (a description of what was happening just before the behaviour occurred), the *behaviour* (a description of the behaviour that occurred) and the *consequences* (what happened after the person engaged in the behaviour).

Mary is a 72-year-old lady living in a care home. She is sitting in a chair in the lounge of the care home. She says in a loud voice, "I need to go, I need to go", gets up from her chair, leaves the lounge and starts to walk down the corridor, all the time saying, "I need to go, I need to go". Her pace quickens and her voice becomes louder.

This has been happening for the past three weeks. Mary becomes very distressed, staff don't understand why this is happening and have been unable to find ways to reduce her distress. She is referred to a specialist team who ask the staff to complete ABC charts.

There are many challenges when using ABC charts. Staff don't know in advance when Mary will become distressed and start walking the corridor. She may start walking and staff may not have observed what was happening before she began to walk (the antecedent). If staff had been observing they would have recorded that Mary was sitting in her chair with four other residents in the lounge, the lounge was relatively quiet and Mary suddenly started to say, "I need to go, I need to go", got up from her chair and left the room. What would staff record as the antecedent – *Mary was sitting in the lounge with four other residents*. The behaviour – *Mary began to say, "I need to go, I need to go", got out of her chair and started to walk the corridor, appearing to be distressed*. The consequence was that *staff approached Mary and invited her to come back to the lounge and sit down*. Did this help? No, Mary continued to walk the corridor and her distress increased.

The ABC charts will continue to be completed each time Mary engages in this behaviour. When there are a few instances, the staff, with the support of the specialist team, will try to understand what may be causing the behaviour and what might help.

As this example highlights, it can be very difficult for staff to know what the antecedent(s) to a behaviour is. Also, when we are involved in a situation we cannot view the situation objectively. We interpret the situation from our own perspective. As a consequence, our opinion of what the antecedent is may not be entirely accurate, it is our simply our opinion. Another person with a different perspective may believe that the antecedent is different. We see examples of this in our life. Two people attend the same event and have different interpretations. They may be talking about the same event but describe it differently, it can sound as if they were not at the same event. One may have enjoyed it and give a positive description with examples of what happened, the other may give a negative description with different examples. Their interests and past experiences influence how they perceive and remember the experience.

Even describing the behaviour is open to interpretation. Often behaviours are recorded as agitation, pacing and verbal or physical aggression. This is an interpretation of the behaviour rather than a description. There is a difference between pacing the corridor and walking along the corridor. Pacing may be the result of agitation but walking may be to get exercise or to go somewhere. One person may interpret a behaviour as aggressive but someone else who sees the same behaviour may not interpret it as aggressive. When we consider the example of John in Chapter 5, the behaviour is waving his stick. Staff may have interpreted this as physical aggression but John's intention was to attract attention.

In addition to the inherent problems of identifying the antecedent, behaviour and consequence, there are practical issues with completing these charts. Timely completion of ABC charts is not always possible. Care homes are busy places and there are multiple demands on staff time. If there is a situation to deal with and a resident is distressed, staff's priority is to deal with this situation and the distress. It may not always be possible to complete an ABC chart during or immediately after an event. If charts are not completed at the time, some of the detail is likely to be omitted. When we rely on our memory of what happened, this is not always accurate, particularly if it was a stressful event. On occasion, ABC charts are completed by a member of staff who did not directly observe the behaviour. At the end of a shift, the behaviour is discussed and a chart is completed. While this demonstrates a willingness of staff to provide as much information as possible, this introduces the potential for inaccurate recording. There are also potential issues of communication, and for some staff, English may not be their first language.

There is a significant degree of training and experience required to recognise antecedents, behaviour, and consequences. Completing the ABC chart requires paying attention to all that is happening in the environment at the time. It is not possible in all care homes to train all staff to ensure they have the necessary experience and expertise to identify the ABCs and accurately complete the chart. As a result, there are some concerns about the quality and reliability of using ABC charts as a tool to help understand behaviour.

To fully understand the meaning of a person's behaviour, we need to see the world from the perspective of that person (Kitwood 1997) and to ascertain when particular behaviours happen. In a care home, staff are with the person for most of the time so it is important to find ways to help staff to accurately record when the behaviour happens.

To get a good understanding of the life of a person with dementia you need to spend time engaging with them and observing their interactions with others. To get a real sense of what someone's life is like you would need to observe them for an extended period of time. This is not always possible and is not an efficient use of resources for a specialist team. You need to enlist the support of care staff who are there all day with the person. You also need to be realistic in the expectations of what care staff can do as they are already very busy. They need to be your eyes in the care home to provide you with enough information to help you to gather the clues that will help to understand behaviour.

CLEAR Dementia Care© Behaviour Record Charts are used to provide information on what someone is doing throughout the day. They record specific behaviours of the person with dementia and this information helps us to understand their behaviour in the context of their environment.

They do not require the person recording the behaviour to interpret the behaviour. They can be completed very quickly by any member of staff. They might record what the behaviour is, for example "S" (shouting), and where it is happening, for example "L" (lounge). Based on the specific behaviours relevant to the individual, care staff agree what codes are most appropriate and recording the behaviour simply requires writing the code (numbers/letters) in a chart. Charts are divided into short time intervals for each day of one week. Often staff will choose codes such as pacing, verbal or physical aggression. When there is a better understanding of the behaviour, the behaviour can be re-labelled as, for example, needing exercise, a change of environment, something to do or misunderstanding the situation.

When the relevant information has been collected, the recordings are colour coded, with a particular behaviour in a particular environment allocated a colour. This facilitates the identification of patterns in behaviour. For some care staff, if there is a behaviour that they find particularly challenging it can feel as if it is happening all the time. Accurate recording provides information about the frequency of specific behaviours. The charts also help care staff to see specific behaviours in context. They can reveal how the activity within the care home throughout the day may impact on a person's behaviour. This is a simple but powerful tool.

The information can be used more specifically to target observation or further recording as appropriate. Sometimes a specialist team will be asked for advice on a person with dementia and as part of the assessment they will complete an observation.

In many cases, the behaviour will not present during the observation and the team may need to return on a number of occasions before they can observe a particular behaviour. The Behaviour Record Charts help to identify when a behaviour is most likely to occur and therefore when it is most appropriate to complete an observation.

When staff recognise patterns in behaviour it helps them to think about what else may have been happening at that time. For example, a person may be distressed in the morning during personal care. Another person may be distressed in the afternoon when the care home is busier with visitors. Care staff start to see the behaviour in the context of the environment and have a greater understanding of the behaviour from the perspective of the person with dementia.

George's chart shows that he is aggressive in the mornings and evenings. George's dementia means that he doesn't have insight into the fact that he needs support with personal care. He resists support from staff, which is initially interpreted by staff as aggression because of his dementia. Edna becomes agitated in the afternoons. She follows staff, seeking reassurance, or she paces the corridor with an anxious expression. Edna gets more confused in busy, noisy environments and starts to feel scared. When visitors arrive in the afternoon, Edna leaves the lounge looking for the safety of staff and walks the corridor as a means of managing her anxiety.

The Behaviour Record Charts give staff greater ownership for understanding behaviour and developing appropriate strategies to reduce distress. They are not relying on an expert to come in to tell them what is going on. They have a good understanding about what is happening in the care home throughout the day.

Staff may need to change their approach to George in the mornings and evenings. Staff may need to support Edna to find a quieter area of the care home before visitors arrive or help her to engage in an activity in her room during the visiting time.

The Behaviour Record Charts help us to see what a typical day is like for the person with dementia. We can then start to think about what it might feel like to have this have this type of day. This opens up potential conversations about how the day could be different. This is important because it is more likely that the care staff will have to change their behaviour as the person with dementia may not be able to change their behaviour. The Behaviour Record Charts help staff to understand why change is important, and when they change their behaviour, it is very likely that as a consequence the behaviour of the person with dementia will also change.

When changes have been implemented, a further Behaviour Record Chart can be completed to monitor the situation. This is also important for staff because it helps to highlight how the changes they have made have had an impact on the quality of life for the person they are caring for.

Care staff have very busy jobs, with multiple demands placed on their time. When we ask them to record behaviour we need to ask them to do something that is manageable within their other work commitments. Behaviour Record Charts provide a good solution as they are quick and easy to fill in and don't require training to complete.

Chapter 7

WHAT DO PEOPLE WITH DEMENTIA NEED?

What do people want out of life? Most people want to be healthy, happy, independent and make their own decisions. People with dementia are no different. There are a number of things we need to enable us to achieve these things.

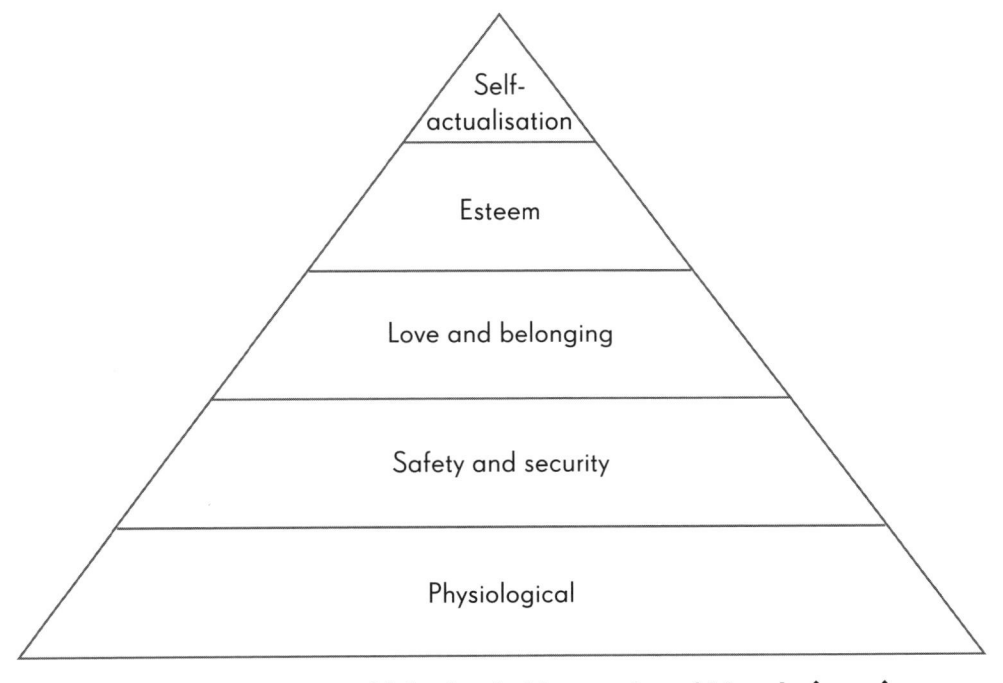

Figure 7.1: A representation of Maslow's Hierarchy of Needs (1943)

Maslow described a hierarchy of needs (Maslow 1943, see Figure 7.1). He proposed that we have to fulfil these needs to be happy. If we don't have our needs met this can impact on our physical and psychological wellbeing. These needs are important to everyone, whether they have a diagnosis of dementia or not. The challenge for a person with dementia is that they may have to depend on others to help meet their needs.

We need to fulfil our basic needs at the bottom of the hierarchy before we move up to the areas at the top of the hierarchy. The needs at the bottom are more physical needs and as we move up the triangle the needs become more psychological and social. Failure to satisfy our needs can have a significant negative impact on our quality of life.

There are basic physiological needs are that are vital to our survival, including air, food, water, clothing, shelter, warmth and sleep. To feel well we need to have enough to eat and drink, have clothes to wear and a place to live and get good sleep.

Most people with dementia have their physiological needs met. However, there are times when it can be difficult to support a person with their physiological needs, for example if they decline to take their meals or their medication. It is easier to identify when physical needs are not being met and then to plan to find ways to meet these needs. If someone is not eating, you could try to offer them different foods or prepare the foods differently. You could also look at where they eat to see if this makes a difference.

As we move further up the hierarchy it can be more difficult for carers to recognise whether the more social and psychological needs are being met. The need for safety and security. What makes us feel safe and secure? It may be recognising the people around you and knowing that they are not going to harm you, or knowing that your belongings are safe. Familiar surroundings may help you to feel safe. Or it may be knowing that you have enough money to look after yourself and your family. The feeling of safety and security is not always something that you can see from the outside so it can be difficult to know whether another person feels safe. We may have to look for clues in a person's behaviour.

If you have impaired memory and you don't know where you are or who the other people around you are, would you feel safe and secure? Sometimes a person with dementia will walk around with all their belongings in a bag. Other people may not understand why they are doing this. Some may think they are paranoid and worried that someone is going to steal from them. Is this paranoia or a normal reaction to their situation? They may regularly misplace things and are living with people they don't know and may assume that their belongings are not safe. If we were in an unfamiliar place with people we didn't know, we would keep our belongings safely with us. When we travel, for example, we are attentive to where our bags are. For some people living with dementia, much of the time they may feel that their belongings are unsafe.

Spending time in a place that is familiar and comfortable to you with people that you know can help you to feel safe. Depending on the stage of their dementia, the people and the surroundings may not be familiar to the person. If we understand that the person may be feeling unsafe then we can care for them in a way that helps them to feel safer. Introducing yourself, telling the person who you are in a friendly tone and giving them time to understand can help. A predictable routine can also help. Remember that in care homes the staff and residents can change frequently and this can have an impact on how safe someone feels. We have to remind ourselves that these vulnerable people with dementia are living 24 hours a day, seven days a week with staff and other residents that they do not know. Having a routine and some control over what happens and when it happens can help them to feel more secure.

Our social needs include love, acceptance and belonging. Emotional relationships are important to all of us. This includes friendships, romantic attachments, family, social groups, community groups, churches and religious organisations. Chapter 3 highlights that people with dementia can lose many of the opportunities for love and social interaction that are so important. Loss of these relationships and social interactions means that there can be an unmet need for love and belonging. It is important to find ways to maintain these relationships or, if this is not possible, to help the person to experience love and belonging from other relationships they do have. This can be communicated by how we engage with the person. Does the person feel valued? When we engage with the person, is it mostly when we support them with personal care or to eat, or are there other times when we engage with them just to spend time talking and participating in an activity? What would life be like if the only time you engaged with someone was when they were supporting you to wash, dress or eat?

Do people with dementia have the opportunity to spend time with people who love them and care about? Do they feel loved and valued? When they try to talk to someone or ask a question, how does that person respond? Do other people take the time to understand what they are saying and respond or do they walk away because they think they have no time or they don't understand what the person is saying?

Esteem is our self-esteem, our confidence, sense of achievement, the respect we feel for others and the respect we receive from others. How do people with dementia experience esteem? Do they feel confident throughout their day? As dementia progresses, the person is likely to feel less confident in their ability to complete most tasks and activities of daily living. How we support the person to compensate for areas of weakness can have a positive or negative impact on their experience. Chapter 4 describes the impact that opportunities to achieve can have on self-esteem. Do you have respect for the people with dementia that you know or care for? Do they feel respected by you? Have you ever talked about the person with dementia when they were in the room and not included them in the conversation? Do you think they would have felt respected if this happened? There are many small things we can do when we engage with a person with dementia which can increase their self-esteem or make them feel worthless. If we treat people with dementia the way we would like to be treated or the way we would treat our mother or father then they are likely to feel loved and respected. Supporting them to do activities which they enjoy and are good at will also have a positive impact on self-esteem.

At the top of the hierarchy is self-actualisation. This is the need to be all that you can be, achieving your full potential without experiencing prejudice. While there are times in our life when we feel that we are achieving our full potential, there are other times when we don't feel that we have the opportunity to do this. Do people living with dementia have the opportunity to experience self-actualisation? Do they have the opportunity to achieve their full potential and live without prejudice? It is not clear that this is the case for all people with dementia.

There is no reason why a person with dementia cannot fulfil their full potential but, in reality, this is not the experience of most people with dementia. There is a tendency to take over, to think, "It's faster if I do it for them", "They can't do it", "They will make too many mistakes", "They might get hurt", "They might break something". What is it like when you feel you have nothing to offer and are not fulfilling your full potential?

Many people with dementia experience stigma. Stigma means that other people have negative assumptions about a particular group or person. Stigma occurs because of a lack of understanding. When you know more about dementia and the person, you realise that these negative assumptions are incorrect and the stigma reduces. CLEAR Dementia Care© helps us to look beyond the label of dementia to see the whole person. When we do this, we can support the person to fulfil their full potential, to fulfil the same needs as everyone else. Why should people with dementia expect anything less?

PART 2

IMPLEMENTING THE CLEAR DEMENTIA CARE© MODEL

Chapter 8

DOMAINS OF CLEAR DEMENTIA CARE©

All behaviour is a form of communication and is often driven by need. Many people with dementia may not be able to tell us what they are thinking, what they want or what they need. For us to really understand their behaviour we need to consider all of the factors that may be contributing to their behaviour. CLEAR Dementia Care© details five domains or areas of life that are important to consider and will help us to understand why a person behaves the way they do (see Figure 8.1).

Cognition: This refers to thinking processes. It includes paying attention learning new things, remembering, talking and understanding language and problem solving. Different types of dementia impact on cognition in different ways (see Chapter 2).

Life story and personality: Looking beyond the label of dementia and interpreting the behaviours in the context of the person's life history and personality is essential. This includes family history, relationships, significant events, previous occupation, hobbies, interests and likes and dislikes. All of these things impact on how a person behaves. This information can also be used to help identify activities that the person may enjoy.

Emotional and physical wellbeing: A person's emotional and physical wellbeing will impact on their behaviour(s) and quality of life.

Activity and environment: How a person spends a typical day and the opportunity to engage in meaningful and appropriate activity impact on behaviour, as do the level of support they need with personal care and activities of daily living, noise, the opportunity for privacy and recent changes in their environment.

Relationships: The quality of a person's relationships with other people is important to how they feel and behave. Good relationships with family, staff and other residents have a positive impact on quality of life. Changes in relationships can have an impact on behaviour.

Support to assess the impact of the five domains is provided in the Aide Memoire to Help Understand Behaviour (see Appendix 2) and Domains Checklist (see Appendix 3).

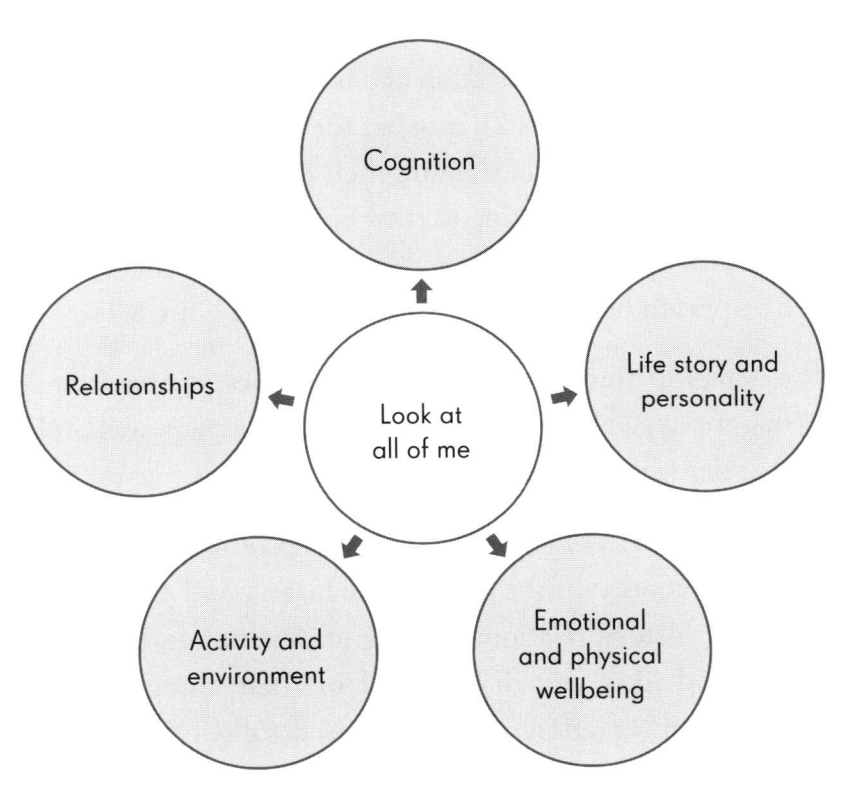

Figure 8.1: CLEAR Dementia Care© Model
© Northern Health and Social Care Trust 2018

COGNITION

Different dementias damage different parts of the brain so different people can be affected in different ways. The person cannot control the effects of this damage. For each person, the type of dementia and the stage of their dementia will determine how their thoughts, feelings and behaviour are affected.

ORIENTATION

Orientation to time, place and person can be impaired. A person may be confused about the time of day, date or year, where they are or who other people are. Whether a person is oriented to time, place and person will determine how they feel, how they respond to others and how others should engage with them.

Orientation to time

There can be confusion about day and night and the person may get up in the night believing it is day time. This can be difficult for carers. Daytime naps and reduced activity can make it harder to sleep at night. Ensuring that there is good light during the day, access to a range of activities, including physical activity and fresh air, will engage the person and help them to sleep. Caffeine in the evening should be avoided. Relaxing in the evening surrounded by familiar things can help. A consistent routine, doing the same things in the same order at the same time will reduce the confusion and distress.

A person may also get mixed up with the time, thinking it is time for breakfast when they have recently had breakfast. They may say that they haven't seen a family member in some time when in fact the relative may have visited very recently. If the person doesn't remember, gentle reminding may help. If the person says, "I haven't seen John for weeks" you could respond by saying, "When John visited last week he told us about his new job." If the person still fails to recall, further reminding may only add to their confusion and distress. Instead ask, "Do you miss John?" or "Shall we ask John to call this week?" If the person is talking about John this means they are thinking about him and may be missing him. Spending some time talking about John may help.

Does the person know what year it is and what age they are, or do they believe that they are younger and have young children to look after or a job to go to? If the person does not recall that they are 80 years old and living in a care home, they may become very distressed when staff stop them from "leaving to go to work". Reminding them that they are aged 80 and living in a care home may add to their confusion and distress. Looking for patterns in the times the person wants to leave for work can help to identify strategies to reduce the distress that can result from this. Generally, if a person is occupied they will be less likely express the need to leave and go to work. The unmet need may be meaningful occupation and purpose. Addressing this may make it less likely that the person wants to leave.

Orientation to place

Does the person know where they are living? If they are living in their own home, do they recognise this to be their home? If they are living in a care home, do they know this and do they know why there are in a care home? A person who no longer recognises their surroundings may feel very anxious about where they are. They may ask to go home, even though they are at their permanent residence. Home is a place where we feel comfortable, safe and secure. When a person living with dementia asks to go home when they are in their permanent residence, this may suggest that they are feeling anxious or unsafe. Chapter 3 discussed that home is not necessarily a building, home can be a feeling – comfort, familiarity, safety and security.

Think about a time when you have been away from a place you call home and you were feeling alone, possibly physically unwell or missing home. Was it the building you were missing? It's more likely to be what that building represented, possibly the family and friends associated with that place. You wanted to be with people who knew you, who would offer you comfort and support. If you weren't able to go home, what did you do? You may have telephoned family or friends, visited a friend or asked a friend to visit you. What may have helped you to feel better was the contact with other people, feeling cared for, feeling that you weren't on your own and you were going to be ok.

This is no different from what a person with dementia experiences when they want to go home. If we understand this then we can think of things that might help. Telling them that they are at home is unlikely to reduce their anxiety. What is likely to help is to sit with them, talk to them, and ask if they need something. Ask them if they are missing someone from home. Looking through some family photographs and reminiscing may help the person to experience familiarity, connection and to feel safe and secure, and they may be less likely to want to leave.

Orientation to person

As dementia progresses, facial recognition and memories fade and the person may no longer recognise family, friends and carers.

What would you do if you were sitting in your living room and a stranger walked in and came towards you? You would most likely be frightened. Who are they? What do they want? How did they get in here? Are they going to harm me? When a person with dementia fails to recognise staff, family or friends, they could potentially be frightened. When you approach them, say hello. If they don't recognise you, tell them who you are. Spend a few minutes talking to them to help them to feel safe. If they still don't recognise you, don't continue to try to get them to understand. Talking to the person in a respectful way, showing them that you care can be enough. For family and friends, showing a picture of you together in the past, or singing a song which may trigger happy memories may elicit a feeling of familiarity and help the person to feel safe. Even if they still don't remember who you are, the photograph may help them to reminisce about your relationship. The interaction may help them to feel safe.

It can be very difficult for families if the person doesn't recognise the person. But, the way you engage with them will let the person know that you are someone who cares for them and they are safe. Trying to remind them who you are may add to their distress. It will be more helpful for the person and for you to enjoy the time you spend without focusing on whether they recognise what your relationship is. The relationship is still important, particularly if the person feels loved and cared for.

SPEED OF PROCESSING

Processing speed is the pace at which you take in information, make sense of it and begin to respond to it. This can be information that you see and hear or movement that you sense. If we say too many things at once it can be confusing for the person, for example, "I'm going to help you get washed and dressed and after breakfast we can go for a walk." A person with slowed processing speed will not follow all of this.

We need to give them more time and break the information down into manageable chunks:

"Shall I help you to get washed?"

"Let's put on your blouse."

"Shall I walk with you to get breakfast?"

ATTENTION AND CONCENTRATION

As you are reading this book, there are many sights, sounds and sensations going on around you: the pressure of your feet against the floor, other objects in the room, the material of your clothing, the memory of a conversation you had earlier in the day. All of these are competing for your attention, but you cannot focus on all of them at the same time. When you try to focus your attention on something, you have to ignore all the other things that are going on at the same time. It can be difficult to focus your attention to engage in conversation or an activity in a busy noisy environment. This can be even more difficult for a person with dementia.

Our ability to stay focused and maintain attention on a task also depends on how interested we are in the task. If we are not interested it is difficult to maintain our attention. Our interest also depends on whether we understand the task or what is being said in the conversation. If you are not interested in what is being said, your mind wanders to something else. Equally, if someone is talking about a topic that you know little about and find difficult to understand, your attention can wander. A person with dementia who is given a task that they don't understand or that is too difficult will not be able to maintain their attention on it. The same is true in conversation; if the pace is too quick or there are long sentences, the person may be unable to keep up so they lose interest and stop paying attention. If a task is too easy, you can become bored and it is hard to maintain your attention. Activities offered need to be appropriate to the person's ability. If they are too hard or too easy the person will have difficulty maintaining attention.

When speaking to a person with dementia we need to ensure that we have their attention. Use their name to make sure the person knows you are talking to them. Make sure they can understand what you are saying, as it will make it easier to pay attention. Use short, simple sentences and give the person enough time to process what you have said.

Divided attention is the ability to engage in two activities at the same time, for example walking and talking. We regularly have a conversation with someone as we walk but some people with dementia find it difficult to walk and talk at the same time. If you are walking with the person and want to engage them in conversation, you may need to stop walking before you expect them to be able to engage effectively in conversation.

MEMORY

Why does memory fail in dementia? The reason for the memory failure can depend on the type of dementia and the stage of the dementia. A person with dementia can experience difficulty with memory because of failure to encode the experience, retrieve the experience or store the experience.

Encoding information into memory

If a person has sensory difficulties and does not hear what is being said or see what is happening then the information will not be encoded in their brain (see section on sensory impairment below). Even with good hearing or sight, if the person is not listening or looking, they will not hear what is being said or see what is happening and it will not be encoded in their brain. We have to be paying attention to the information for it to be processed by our brain. It is important to check that the person with dementia knows that you are talking to them and they are listening. We also need to understand the information to encode it. If the information was not encoded, we cannot say that it has been forgotten because it was never processed. If the information has been attended to and encoded, it then has to be successfully stored in memory.

Storing information as a memory

Events and experiences need to be successfully stored in memory to enable us to recall the experience at a later time. In some dementias, the part of the brain responsible for storing memories, the hippocampus, part of the temporal lobe, is damaged. People often ask, "How can she remember what happened 30 years ago but can't remember what happened ten minutes ago?" Events and experiences that happened before the dementia are already stored in the brain so these memories already exist. This is why the person with dementia may be able to remember things that happened years ago. New memories need to be created and stored. If the ability to store information is impaired then new events, conversations and experiences will be forgotten. If a person asks, "When are we having dinner?" and you respond, "Remember, we had dinner an hour ago, it was fish and potatoes?" this will not help the person with Alzheimer's disease to remember because the experience of having dinner was not stored in memory so it is as if it never happened.

As dementia progresses and more parts of the brain are damaged, information and experiences that were stored in the brain before the dementia gradually disappear. The person may no longer be able to remember events that happened ten or more years ago. Even reminding the person will not help them to remember as the information has been lost from their brain.

Retrieving a memory

If an event or experience has been stored in our memory, we need to be able to retrieve that information later. Sometimes memories are stored in our brain but we just can't retrieve them – this is called retrieval failure. With the right prompt or clue sometimes the memories come back. We've all experienced hearing a song that is associated with our past and with the song come many memories associated with that time. The same can be true for a picture or a smell. Going back to a place from your younger days triggers memories that you thought you had forgotten. The memories were still stored in your brain but you hadn't retrieved them.

Sometimes if you have forgotten, clues can help. When you recognise a face but cannot remember the name, you think about where you know the person from to see if that will jog your memory. Sometimes you go through the alphabet to try to jog your memory: A – Alex, B – Brian, C – Clive, D – David, yes, it's David! The tip of the tongue experience is another example of retrieval failure. You know the word you are looking for but you just can't get it. This can be a very frustrating experience. Sometimes you need lots of clues to help you remember. "Remember when we went to the park and met Jane; she was with her husband Robert…"

In the earlier stages, a person with vascular dementia may be able to store new experiences in memory. They may later appear to have forgotten because, while the experience is stored in memory, they may be unable to retrieve the memory. For example, if you ask a person with vascular dementia, "When did Brian visit?" they may respond with,

"I don't know." If you prompt them by asking, "Did you enjoy seeing Brian last night and hearing about his new job?" this may be enough to jog their memory and they may respond, "Yes, I did, he brought me a lovely bunch of flowers." Prompting with some information can trigger the recall of the memory. However, prompting is unlikely to help a person with Alzheimer's disease as the memory will not have been stored.

Types of memory

We have different types of memory and different parts of the brain are involved in these different types of memory. What the person can and cannot remember depends on the parts of the brain that are affected by dementia. The two main types of memory are short-term memory and long-term memory (Atkinson and Shiffrin 1968). Within long-term memory there are three types: episodic memory, semantic memory and procedural memory (Tulving 1985).

Short-term memory

Short term memory is the ability to hold information for a short period of time. When you look up a phone number and begin to dial the number, the number is held in short-term memory. When you have dialled the number and stopped paying attention to it, you will quickly forget it because the information was only held in short-term memory. When we are having a conversation, we rely on our short-term memory to remember what the person has just said to enable us to respond.

In conversation, a person with dementia may respond appropriately because they can hold the conversation in short-term memory. If you leave the room and come back a short time later, they may not remember what was said or even that you had a recent conversation. The person has preserved short-term memory but they are not storing this information in long-term memory. For example, a person with dementia may ask, "When are we going to the doctor?" and you respond, "The appointment is at 4 o'clock." Ten minutes later the person asks, "When are we going to the doctor?" A person with Alzheimer's disease has no recollection that ten minutes ago you told them what time the appointment was. They have failed to store this information in long-term memory because the part of the brain which stores this information, the hippocampus in the temporal lobe, is not working properly. It is as if they were never told the information.

Long-term memory

There are different types of long-term memory which are responsible for the recognition of everyday objects (semantic memory), recall of recent events (episodic memory), and remembering how to do things (procedural memory).

Semantic memory is our general knowledge of the world; for example, knowing that a cat is an animal, a cup is something that we use to drink from and Paris is the capital of France. We don't need to remember when or where we learned this information to know the information. If semantic memory is impaired, the person may fail to recognise everyday objects.

Episodic memory is our memory for a particular event or experience at a particular time – the ability to recall events, for example that your sister visited the day before or when you were aged 16 years you secured your first part-time job in a shop. It is the ability to remember where you have put things or whether you have taken your medication.

Sometimes family and friends might think, "What's the point in visiting because they don't recognise me and won't remember the visit?" There is every point. The person may not recognise you or may not recall that you have visited but they can enjoy a positive experience while you are there. The person may not understand all that you are saying but they will recognise the emotion. Your tone and body language can make the person feel safe, cared for and loved. When you leave, they may not remember details of the visit but they will remember how you made them feel. This positive emotion may remain for longer than the visit. All of these positive experiences add up to significantly improving a person's quality of life.

Procedural memory is our memory for skills, for example your ability to swim, ballroom dance or ride a bicycle. It is very difficult to describe how we do these things and you can best demonstrate your memory by actually doing them.

Dementia can cause impairment in one or more of these types of memory and as the dementia progresses all types of memory are affected.

LANGUAGE

Dementia can make it hard for people to communicate, and this can be upsetting and frustrating for the person and for those around them. Language difficulties can be present in both the ability to express what they want to say and to understand what other people are saying. The person may be unable find the right words and this can make it difficult for them to tell us what they want. They may substitute the wrong word, such as "book" instead of "newspaper" use non-words, for example "papple" for "apple", or use substitutes like "thing to sit on" instead of "chair", or they may not be able to find any words to tell us what they want.

Sometimes the person will not understand what you have said and will reply in conversation with something that is unrelated to what you have been talking about. Some people have speech that is fluent but doesn't have any meaning, for example they may use jumbled up words and grammar. This can cause frustration and confusion for both the person and those around them and can lead to tension.

We take for granted that we use language to communicate with other people. We talk to others about our day and ask about their day. The ability to communicate is an important part of our social life. Think about your day and how often you communicate with other people. How well we can do this impacts on our quality of life. If someone misinterprets what we have said, this is frustrating and, depending on the circumstances, can lead to increased stress.

If you want help with something or need something, you use language to ask. What would it be like if you were unable to tell people what you wanted? If you have been in a country where you don't speak the language, it can be a real challenge to go about your day. Sometimes you have to be creative, using gestures to try to communicate what you want.

We also use language to express our wishes and feelings. If you couldn't do any of this, what would your life be like?

The person with dementia may not understand all of what you are saying but they will understand your emotion. How you engage with them can help them to feel safe and respected. People with dementia may no longer be able to find words but they do still have thoughts and feelings which they will try to communicate. We need to take time to recognise, respect and respond to them. Patient, respectful, caring communication continues to be important for all people with dementia, no matter what stage of dementia they are at.

When supporting a person with dementia it is better to give positive instructions, for example instead of saying, 'Don't go there' say, 'Shall we go here?' Involve the person in conversation and listen. Be aware that the person's reasoning and logic may be affected by dementia. Arguing, disagreeing or correcting may only lead to frustration.

If someone is not able to express themselves effectively, they can lose confidence, or feel anxious, depressed or withdrawn. Following and engaging in conversation can be difficult and tiring. This can lead to a normally outgoing person becoming quieter, more introverted and less interested in social interaction. The person may also behave in ways that we find difficult to understand because they are trying to communicate what they can no longer say with words. Behaviour is a form of communication.

Like all of us, people with dementia will reflect the mood of those around them. How you approach and communicate with them will impact on their response.

Reading and writing can also be impaired. Many people get great pleasure from reading books, newspapers, magazines, letters, emails or test messages from friends. No longer being able to engage in these activities is a significant loss and can have a very negative impact on the person.

VISUOSPATIAL PROCESSING

Visuospatial processing is our ability to understand what we see, what size it is and where it is. Dementia can cause damage to the brain's ability to process the information that the eye receives. It may appear to be a sight problem but is not caused by an eye condition.

Impairment in visuospatial processing can impact on many activities of daily living. When reaching for a cup to drink from, the person may misjudge the distance and reach past the cup. When eating, it can be difficult to accurately locate the food on the plate or accurately move the food from the plate to the mouth to eat it. This may cause people to only eat part of what is on their plate. Impaired visuospatial processing can also cause the person to frequently drop objects or spill food and drinks.

Getting dressed can be more difficult because of visuospatial impairment, locating the appropriate clothing and judging the co-ordinated movement to put clothing on. Dressing can also be impaired because of problems in sequencing.

Dementia can affect depth perception and the ability to see objects in three dimensions. This makes it more difficult to go down stairs and increases the risk of falls. Getting in and out of the bath or the car can be more difficult. The person can have problems judging how far away things are and can become clumsy or bump into things.

They may become disoriented and confused about where they are, become lost or unable to find their way home from a place they have previously known well, or be unable to find the bathroom in the middle of the night. Recognising familiar faces or locating familiar objects which are in plain sight, for example finding milk in the fridge, can become more difficult.

The ability to read may also decline, in part due to visuospatial changes as well as a decline in ability to remember how to read or comprehend the meaning of the words, as discussed earlier.

Peripheral vision may be impaired, and if you approach the person from the side they may not see you coming. It will seem as if you have suddenly appeared from nowhere and this can be very frightening. If this happens, the person may lift their hand to protect themselves from this sudden object appearing in front of them. This can then be misinterpreted as aggression. If you approach slowly from the front, the person is more likely to see you coming. Say hello as you approach to attract their attention.

Some people may eat from other people's plates as they may not be able to see the plate in front of them but can see the plate of the person sitting opposite. The person does not realise that this is not their plate. This can be interpreted as a deliberate act to take food from another person when it is actually a problem with visual processing.

EXECUTIVE FUNCTION

Executive function can be seen as the control function of the brain. It is the ability to solve problems, sequence, organise and plan. It also includes the ability to control behaviour and emotions. Making decisions, starting a task, monitoring and keeping track of what you are doing and making changes if appropriate are all executive functions.

Many of our activities of daily living require executive functions. Impairment can make it difficult to correctly order the multiple steps required to carry out activities, for example to put on clothing in the correct order when getting dressed.

The sequencing, planning and organising necessary to make a cup of tea or cook a meal can be impaired. Shopping can be difficult – making decisions about what items to buy and then paying for them.

Initiation is the ability to start a task or come up with ideas about what to do. With impaired initiation, it can appear as if the person has "no get up and go". They may seem to lack interest or motivation to do anything or have difficulty starting an activity. A person can also become disinhibited. Inhibition is the ability to stop yourself from saying something or acting in a certain way if it is not appropriate, for example making a negative comment to a person you do not know about their appearance. It is knowing that it is not appropriate to make sexual comments to people you do not know or remove your clothing in public places. It is also the ability to resist temptation. If you have a box of chocolates and are planning to save them for later, to do this, you need to inhibit the urge to eat them now. It is the ability to stop acting impulsively, for example resisting the impulse to buy things that you don't need or cannot afford. Impairment in executive function means that the person may say or do things on impulse without thinking about the consequences.

The ability to shift attention can be impaired. This is the ability to change what you are doing or thinking about when the situation changes. Also, the ability to monitor your performance and decide if you are on track and if not to make changes to what you are doing. This can cause the person to continue to do something in one way, even if it is not working. They are unable to change how they are doing it. Or being unable to cope with change or not being able to see things from another person's point of view. This can cause significant tension as carers try unsuccessfully to persuade the person to do things differently.

Emotional control is the ability to manage your emotions by using rational thought. If you are annoyed about something, you know that it is not appropriate to shout at other people and hit out. Lack of emotional control means that you may over react and become angry or upset about relatively minor things.

Poor judgement and reasoning means that the person may need support to make decisions about health care, finance and accommodation.

AWARENESS

Lack of awareness may arise from a combination of both neuropsychological and psychological reasons. Neuropsychological unawareness occurs because of damage to the brain. The part of the brain which enables a person to be aware of their strengths and weakness is not functioning properly. Psychological unawareness occurs because the person does not acknowledge particular difficulties or minimises the severity and impact they have. Lack of awareness means that the person may not realise they need support. This can be stressful and a source of conflict if not managed sensitively. It can also present a potential risk if the person is not aware that they are no longer safe to complete some activities.

Unawareness

A person can be unaware of the impact of the dementia because the part of the brain that enables them to perceive their strengths and weaknesses is damaged. This is not a psychological denial because the person does not want to come to terms with the consequences of the dementia but is a genuine inability to understand the consequences of the dementia.

For this neurologically based unawareness – anosagnosia – talking about what the person cannot do or drawing attention to areas of weakness will not help the person to see the impact that dementia has on their ability. Highlighting limitations will increase their distress. Changes to your behaviour, the environment and how the support is offered are the most helpful responses.

Denial

Psychological denial is when the person resists accepting the impact dementia is having on their activities of daily living. There can also be denial combined with some unawareness of the extent of impairment.

Uncertainty

Some people experience a state of confusion about the impact of dementia, and what the implications are for their everyday activities. The person can fluctuate between being more optimistic or more pessimistic about what the future holds.

Some people who are more aware of the impact of dementia can experience a range of emotions and respond in different ways, including anger, depression and acceptance.

Anger

The person may not accept that they may have to stop doing some things or change the way they do other things. They can react angrily if someone else tries to impose restrictions on what they can do. Offering support in a way that is acceptable to the person is important. Compromise and some creativity may be needed to explore ways to maximise strengths and find ways to compensate for identified weakness. Dementia requires significant adjustment for the person and for those who care for and support them. Responding to anger in a calm and patient manner can be difficult at times but will stop the anger from escalating.

Depression

Depression is an understandable and common consequence of dementia. Depression is associated with feelings of sadness, hopelessness, worthlessness, and despair. This can be accompanied by loss of interest and motivation, leading to social withdrawal. Fatigue, loss of energy, changes in eating and sleeping patterns are also common. Depression may also present as increased irritability, agitation and aggressiveness. The person may feel out of control and helpless in making decisions about their life and feel dependent on others.

Acceptance

This is when the person accepts the changes that are associated with dementia and adjusts to a new routine and new ways of doing things. Acceptance is easier to achieve if the person has the opportunity to remain as independent as possible with their activities of daily living, and is included as much as possible in decision making. The way care and support are offered can have a significant impact on the acceptance of the changes in ability and the adjustment to these changes.

BEHAVIOUR AND PERSONALITY CHANGES

There are many reasons for changes in behaviour. Changes could result directly from neuropsychological impairments, for example when behaviour is disinhibited and inappropriate in the social setting. Other reasons include changes in interests as dementia progresses, changes in physical wellbeing, misunderstanding situations or lack of meaningful activity. Failure to understand changes in behaviour can cause significant distress for the person and their carers.

MOTOR FUNCTION

Motor impairment can cause apraxia (difficulty planning movements). This can impact on activities of daily living such as the ability to button and unbutton clothes or use utensils to eat. In order to complete accurate movements, the brain tells different parts of the body to work in a co-ordinated way. As dementia progresses these messages become impaired. Ataxia (poor co-ordination and balance) increases the risk of falls. As dementia progresses there is a decline in mobility.

For any activity, many of these cognitive functions are involved. Making a cup of tea is something that most of us do every day. It seems like a very simple task and we do it almost automatically without paying much attention to it. But it is a complex task that requires a range of cognitive functions and many parts of the brain:

- Register that you are thirsty.
- Make a decision that you want tea to quench your thirst.
- Remember what tea is.
- Walk to the kitchen where you make tea.
- Recognise all the items you need, kettle, cup and so on.
- Remember where all these items are kept: cup in cupboard, spoon in drawer and so on.
- Remember the correct sequence: put water in the kettle, boil the kettle, get the cup, tea bag and so on.

You could fail at making tea because of your memory, visuospatial processing, motor processing, executive function or a combination of these. If we understand the reason why the person is unsuccessful, we can support them to do the parts that they cannot do to enable them to be as independent as possible.

HALLUCINATIONS

This is seeing or hearing things that are not there which may cause distress. If someone is having hallucinations it is usually not helpful to try to convince them that what they are seeing or hearing is not there. What the person is experiencing is real to them at the time. Offering reassurance that you are there and they are safe can help. Engaging in an activity to distract from the hallucination may help.

ILLUSIONS

Misinterpretation of what is seen or heard can also occur, for example mistaking a pile of socks for snakes or a wardrobe for the bathroom. Misperceptions can be triggered by excess noise or reflective or patterned surfaces (see the section on sensory impairment). The person may see an animal in a patterned curtain, or see a rug on the floor, but interpret it as a hole in the ground. These can cause significant distress. Check that glasses and hearing aids are up to date and in use.

DELUSIONS

The person may have difficulty understanding what is real from what is imagined. They may believe that something is true that is not true. They may falsely believe that someone is trying to poison them, stealing from them or their partner is having an affair. As discussed in Chapter 2, hallucinations and visual misperceptions may explain some of the delusions people experience. Delusions can be very distressing for the person and those around them. It is usually not helpful to try to convince them that what they believe is not true. Offering reassurance that you are there and they are safe can help.

SLEEP DISTURBANCES

There may be disruption of the sleep wake cycle, for example waking in the middle of the night thinking that it is time to go to work (see above the section on orientation). Chapter 2 describes REM Sleep Disorder, which is common in Lewy body dementia.

DRIVING

In the early stages of dementia the person may still be able to drive but over time their ability to drive will diminish. Driving will become more difficult, in part because of changes in the ability to understand spatial relationships and judge distances. For example, navigating a turn, changing lanes or parking a car could become a significant challenge. Impairment in divided or sustained attention and impulsivity will also have a negative impact on driving.

LIFE STORY AND PERSONALITY

A person with dementia is a person who has lived a life like every other person. The way they live their life now may be different because of the changes in their ability as a result of their dementia. They may not be able to communicate and express themselves as well as they could before, but that doesn't change who they are. That does not change the life they have lived.

Sometimes we can avoid or become anxious around people we do not know. Many people don't understand dementia, what it is, and what it means for that person. When you take this lack of understanding and combine it with a person who has difficulty telling others what it is like to have dementia, the challenge of understanding is greater.

If you didn't know the person before they had dementia you may assume that how they behave now is who they are. For example, if you interpret a person's behaviour as being aggressive, you may believe that "James is an aggressive person". The behaviour is attributed to the person's personality rather than as a direct consequence of what they are feeling at the time, which may be scared and confused.

A better understanding of James and his personality may highlight that he is usually a mild-mannered man and rarely gets cross.

If you don't know anything about a person, it's harder to know how best to talk to them. What would they like to talk about? If you talk, do they understand what you are saying? If you tried to make conversation with someone at work or at a social event and they didn't respond, you would assume they weren't interested. We all have people we enjoy talking to in social situations and other people we tend to avoid because we feel we have less in common with them. How do you know you have something in common with someone? It's because you share your thoughts about things and share something about your life and your history. It's also because you find it easy to talk to them, they seem interested in what you are saying and they respond when you ask a question. You have found some common ground or common interests. If they don't respond, you assume they are not interested.

You may believe that you have nothing in common with a person with dementia if you don't know anything about their life, their interests, likes and dislikes and they are not able to tell you. You may misinterpret that the person with dementia is not interested or does not understand what you are saying. If so, is there any point in talking to them? Yes, there is, but we need to think about what we are saying and how we are saying it. When talking to a person with dementia, it can be harder for them to understand and respond. This makes it more difficult for us. We may need to be more creative in how we communicate and may also have to work hard to understand their response.

Fast forward 20, 40 or 60 years into the future. What if you had dementia? How would you want to be treated? Think of all your achievements, the highs and lows of your life. We all have lived different lives, each of them interesting in their own way. Different people experience different challenges and have different achievements. All our lives are different but that doesn't make any of our lives more or less important, they are all of equal value. How do we show someone that they are valued? Sometimes it is what we say to them but more often it is by how we treat them.

What if someone was caring for you and they didn't know anything about you and assumed that because you didn't communicate that you didn't understand anything. What would that feel like if your past and your achievements were just wiped out and you became just someone who needed to be cared for?

KATE

Kate had a very happy childhood, she enjoyed playing outside. She was described as a tomboy who was always covered in bruises from climbing trees. She met Bill when she was aged 18 years, they fell in love and married. She worked as a care assistant but gave this up when her first child was born and she remained at home until all of her three children, Emma, Ronan and Katie, were at school. One of her children, Ronan, was killed in a road traffic accident aged 5 years. Kate never got over the tragic death of Ronan but she carried on as best she could for the sake of her other two children. When the children were older, Kate became a childminder. She devoted her life to caring for other children; she was very kind and all the children loved her. She looked after her six grandchildren until she was diagnosed with Alzheimer's disease aged 78 years. Kate is much loved by her children, grandchildren and many friends.

What if you were Kate and I look at you but I don't really see you. I support you to get up and dressed but I don't know that pink is your favourite colour and you never liked wearing grey because it was too dull. I support you to eat breakfast but I don't see that you hate porridge and like one sugar in strong tea. I support you to sit in the communal lounge beside people you don't know with the TV on. You can't see the TV because your vision is poor. You would never have watched TV during the day anyway because you always liked to be busy. I look at you but don't see that you have nothing to do now, that there is no purpose to your day. I don't know about how much you loved and were loved and about the heartbreaking loss of your second child, Ronan. I ask you a question but I don't wait for you to answer. At other times when you do answer I don't understand what you are saying so I ignore what you have said.

That life lived and the person, Kate, is still there but I can't see you. I don't see that the dementia hasn't stripped your past, you are still you. What if I no longer see Kate, I just see an 82-year-old lady with dementia? How does that make you feel?

Everyone has an interesting history peppered with challenges and achievements.

It is important that people who know the person with dementia well provide information about that person's life to those who are caring for them – their likes and dislikes and also the challenges and achievements they experienced throughout their life. When we know something about the people we interact with, it changes how we interact with them, how we care for them. They won't be just a person we support with personal care who has dementia. They will be Brian, who worked all his life in the council refuse department and married Barbara, the love of his life. Or Catherine, a great baker who baked cakes for birthdays, weddings and other celebrations. Or Sophie, who loved to dance and will come alive when she hears her favourite music.

It is disrespectful to care for someone and not take the time to get to know who they are. Sharing a life story is one of the most powerful, yet simple ways we can improve the way a person is supported. It changes our approach, how we engage, it brings the person into the room and leaves their dementia at the door.

The life history provides information about the person's previous occupations. When someone is older we can forget that they had a job and we can often be surprised to hear the jobs that people with dementia have had and the lives that they have lived. If someone can't communicate very well we often don't ask ourselves, "What would they have been like before?" Knowing about a person's history makes you think about them differently. It can also can help to understand their behaviour.

BRENDA

Brenda was always going up to other residents and rearranging their clothing or trying to feed them or give them a drink. This often caused altercations with other residents who did not want Brenda to touch them or take their things. Staff thought this was part of the dementia and Brenda's behaviour was labelled as "interfering with other residents". Brenda became upset and confused when other residents declined her help or when staff asked her to stop feeding other residents. When Brenda's family provided information on her life history staff found out that Brenda had been a care worker all her working life. She believed that she was still a care worker and she was offering support to the other residents. When staff understood her behaviour they no longer saw Brenda as causing problems but recognised that she was trying to help. Brenda was given jobs to do around the home. This fulfilled her need to care for others and have purposeful activity. Brenda was much happier and staff felt that their increased understanding of Brenda meant that they could offer her better care. At times, Brenda continued to try to feed other residents but staff no longer saw this as a problem and were able to quickly redirect Brenda to another helping task when she did this.

ROBERT

Robert was always lifting other residents walking frames and tables and moving them into a bathroom. Staff were concerned about this behaviour. Robert was causing a potential risk to other residents when he removed their walking frame. This also caused distress and altercations as some of the residents resisted Robert's attempts to take their walking frame. When staff attempted to stop Robert, he shouted at staff and if they did not move out of his way, he would push past them and carry on with what he was doing. Robert's daughter advised that Robert had worked as a removals man. Staff understood that Robert thought his job was to move the tables and frames and he was storing them in the bathroom. Robert was given jobs to do around the care home to occupy him during the times when he believed that he should be working.

MICHAEL

Michael was urinating behind furniture in the lounge and in corners in the corridors and rooms. Staff found this behaviour difficult to understand and it was causing distress for other residents. Michael had worked in a mobile shop and often found himself needing to go to the toilet along country roads.

On occasion, he would have gone to the toilet behind a hedge. Michael's dementia meant that he was unable to find the toilet in the care home and so was going to the toilet "behind a hedge", which was actually behind furniture or in a corner. Behaviour Record Charts helped to identify when this was more likely to happen. Clear signage was put on the toilet doors and staff proactively supported Michael to go to the toilet at regular times throughout the day.

Understanding a person's life history can help us to understand their behaviour. Knowing what a person's normal routines are is also important.

ANNA

Staff reported that Anna had poor sleep and she was regularly found in her nightwear walking the corridor. Her family advised that Anna had always been an early riser who was up at 5am every morning. When staff were aware of this they were able to support Anna to get up earlier in the morning before the other residents. Anna's behaviour was no longer interpreted as "wandering the corridor". She had woken disoriented and was looking for staff to help her get dressed. Anna enjoyed sitting the in quiet lounge with her rummage bag while staff supported the other residents to get up.

In the same way as previous occupation is important, knowing what someone's role within the family was can help us to get to know the person. Their hobbies, interests, likes and dislikes are also important. Their personality and how they coped with things in the past is also helpful.

CLEAR Dementia Care© recommends that every person with dementia has an Understanding Document. This includes a brief summary of the person's history which helps to show the person beyond the label of their dementia. It contains enough information to give a better understanding of the person but is short enough that all staff who work with the person will have time to read it. It may seem disrespectful to summarise a person's life in such a brief manner, but if there is too much information it is less likely that it will be read. It is in the best interests of the person to provide brief information that everyone can read, than comprehensive information that many of the staff will not have time to read. This is particularly important for new staff and agency staff. More detailed information can be provided in a Life Story book which staff can read when they have more time.

EMOTIONAL AND PHYSICAL WELLBEING
EMOTIONAL WELLBEING

We all feel our moods change from time to time and people with dementia are no different. People with dementia may experience a range of feelings. They may grieve for the loss of their abilities, skills and independence. They may experience anger, denial or helplessness. There is also uncertainty about what is going to happen in the future. How the disease will progress, slowly or quickly, and how it will affect relationships with family and friends, their daily life and plans for the future. They may feel more isolated as their environment becomes unfamiliar and more confusing.

The person may not be able to understand or express how they feel but still may have a general feeling that something is wrong. This may cause anxiety or agitation.

The person may develop apathy – a loss of interest or motivation to start or continue with an activity. They may not be interested in what other people are doing or not want to engage with other people. Apathy can develop because of damage to the frontal lobe of the brain, or it may result from a failure to understand what is happening and a resultant loss of interest.

The person may experience depression in which they feel sad, hopeless or irritable much of the time. For some people, this is because they have difficulty concentrating or remembering. This can cause a loss of self-confidence. Depression can also be a side effect of certain medications.

The symptoms of depression can be similar to the symptoms of dementia so it can be difficult to identify depression. Depression can also make the symptoms of dementia worse. It is important to diagnose depression because it may respond to treatment. Some common symptoms of depression include:

- Loss of interest in previously enjoyed activities or hobbies.
- Lack of energy.
- Problems sleeping.
- Increased confusion.
- Loss of appetite and weight.
- Wanting to spend more time alone or spending more time in their room.

WHAT CAN YOU DO TO HELP?

- Plan for the future, while the person is still able to express their wishes and desires. This can give the person a feeling of control at a time when they might be feeling helpless.
- Focus on what the person can do rather than what they cannot do.
- Establish a consistent daily routine. The predictability will reduce confusion.
- Support them to keep doing the things they enjoy.
- Introduce a small amount of the activity at a time.
- Make sure the activity is appropriate to the person's level of ability, not too easy or too difficult.
- Include a range of activities, including ones that do not require active participation, such as listening to music.
- Support the person to express how they're feeling, if they want to.
- For people who are unable to communicate verbally, use music or creative activities to potentially help them to express how they feel.

People with depression can also experience anxiety and feelings of isolation. This can increase the social isolation already experienced by people with dementia.

Chapter 3 discusses how some of the losses in memory might cause anxiety. A person may be losing things and not have insight that they have dementia. They will not recall where they have put things. They may believe that someone else has moved their things. This could be frustrating, scary or confusing. When we cannot find something that we need, we are frustrated, we may be worried that we will not be able to find it on time or we may worry that it has been permanently lost or stolen. Losing things may lead the person with dementia to believe that people are stealing or hiding things from them. This can increase their anxiety.

Sometimes, a person may lose the ability to control their emotions. There can be rapid mood changes that fluctuate. Or the person may become emotional about what seem like relatively trivial events. This can be difficult for carers and can lead to tension.

We all worry sometimes or feel sad, lonely or stressed. We all have different ways of coping with these experiences. We could talk to a friend or go for a walk. What if you were no longer able to engage in these coping strategies? There is a good chance that you would feel worse. A person with dementia is no different, they will have had their unique way of dealing with life's challenges. Their coping strategies may no longer be available to them. This could be because reduced mobility means they cannot go for a walk or impaired language skills may mean that they cannot tell others how they are feeling. Loss of coping strategies can increase agitation and distress.

Some people will have experienced mental health difficulties before they developed dementia. Knowing how they coped in the past is helpful. Some of the strategies they used may still be helpful. Others may no longer be appropriate. If people have had difficult or traumatic experiences in their past, they may be re-experiencing these difficult or traumatic times. Close attention to what they are saying and how they are behaving, together with knowledge of their life history, can help to understand how they might be feeling and what support may be helpful.

A greater understanding of how the person is feeling can help to identify things that may help. Looking for changes in behaviour and considering all of the other things that are happening around the person can provide the clues to how they might be feeling. Have there been changes to staff or residents that may have increased their anxiety? Have there been changes to the pattern of visitors which may have had an impact on their mood? Has there been a deterioration in their condition which has increased the support they need or means they can no longer take part in activities that they enjoy?

It is important to remember that even in the later stages of dementia, the person is still able to experience a variety of emotions such as joy, love, fear and sadness. How we engage with the person can have a significant impact on how they feel.

PHYSICAL WELLBEING

Many changes in physical health and wellbeing can cause increased confusion and delirium. People with dementia are already confused so knowing when behaviour might be caused by dementia or a change in physical health can be difficult. It is important to monitor changes in physical health if there has been a recent change in the person's behaviour.

PAIN

When we experience pain, we can take steps to alleviate the pain. We can rest, take appropriate medication or seek advice from a medical practitioner if appropriate. We can tell other people that we are in pain and seek comfort and support from family and friends. What about a person with dementia who may not be able to find the words to tell us that they are in pain. How would we know they need to rest, be comforted, receive medication or see a medical practitioner?

Short-term conditions that can cause pain

There are many conditions, such as a headache, that can cause pain which most of the time can be alleviated with appropriate treatment. How do you feel when you have a headache? You may feel grumpier, you may want peace and quiet and to not engage with people as this may make your headache feel worse. You may take pain relief medication. Other examples could be if you twist or turn and pull a muscle or bump into something and hurt yourself. This may cause discomfort when moving or getting in and out of bed. What if you have dementia and you have a headache or a pulled muscle? You experience the same pain but you may not have the language to tell someone how you are feeling. How do you get the medication or let someone know that it is sore to get in and out of bed? How would people know that you just want peace and quiet for a while? If a person with dementia seems a bit more cross with family, friends or carers, how would these people know that they are experiencing pain?

Long-term conditions that can cause pain

As we get older it is more likely that we will develop physical illness or have a long-term physical health condition. Some of these conditions may cause pain and discomfort. With increasing age, people are also more likely to experience stiffness in joints or have arthritis. All of these can make movement more difficult and painful.

How do we respond to pain?

Pain increases our agitation and this is no different for a person with dementia than it is for a person who does not have dementia. If we are supporting a person who is experiencing pain this can be particularly difficult first thing in the morning when they are being moved and supported with personal care. If we fail to understand this we can unintentionally increase the pain they experience, which will increase their distress and agitation. Carers often report verbal and physical aggression when they support a person with dementia with personal care. If we have hurt a part of our body and someone attempts to move or touch that part of the body, our natural reaction is to call out in pain, tell them it is sore and ask them to stop or move to defend ourselves from the movement to stop the pain. If this is happening to a person with dementia and they are not able to tell us they are in pain, we will not understand when they cry out or act in a way to stop us from hurting them. We may misinterpret their calling out or their attempts to stop us from hurting them as verbal or physical aggression.

When we understand the other person's perspective we can do things differently. If we know that the person has a condition which may cause pain with movement, we can make sure they are given prescribed pain relief and it has had time to take effect before we attempt to support them to move. We could also think about how we support them to move, to reduce the potential impact of pain. We could engage with them in a way that they are distracted and so less focused on the pain they experience. Sometimes singing a song with someone during personal care can help the person to relax. When they are engaged and paying attention to the music, the experience of pain can be reduced.

If a person's behaviour changes, we need to consider whether they may be experiencing pain. Resistance to support with personal care as a result of pain is common, especially first thing in the morning. This resistance can be misinterpreted by carers as aggression. Throughout the day, restlessness, agitation and calling out are all common responses to being in pain.

INFECTION

Older adults are more susceptible to infection, which can also be harder to recognise in people with dementia. This can lead to ongoing discomfort.

There are many types of infections, but the most common types are respiratory infection and urinary tract infection (UTI). Older adults are at increased risk of respiratory infections because of changes in lung capacity and other physical health conditions such as cardiopulmonary disease or diabetes. As dementia progresses, it may be harder to maintain personal hygiene, for example washing regularly and changing clothes. This may increase the risk of developing a UTI. Also, people with a weak immune system with diabetes are at greater risk of a UTI.

If the person is unable to tell you how they feel, it is important to be familiar with the symptoms of infection and seek advice from the person's GP to ensure they get the correct treatment. Symptoms that may be consistent with infection include loss of appetite, decline in the ability to do things they could normally do, change in mood, change in behaviour, increased confusion, fatigue, incontinence and falls. While some of these symptoms may be present in many people with dementia, the key is where there has been a recent change.

Infection can also trigger a delirium.

DELIRIUM

Delirium is the sudden onset of an acute confusional state which usually develops over a few hours or a few days. It is caused by a number of conditions, such as a severe or chronic medical illness, changes in metabolic balance (such as low sodium), medication, infection or surgery.

People with dementia are at greater risk of developing delirium and the risk increases when in hospital or living in a care home. The symptoms of delirium and dementia can be similar but family and carers will notice a change in how the person is and find that the person is "not themselves".

It is important to treat delirium as a medical emergency. Medical staff can identify and treat the cause of the delirium. Prompt treatment will help the person get better and avoid medical complications. It will also reduce distress for the person and those who care for them.

Symptoms

Symptoms of delirium include increased confusion that can fluctuate throughout the day. There may also be periods when there are no symptoms. Symptoms also tend to be worse during the night when it is dark and things look less familiar.

Reduced awareness of the environment

The person may:

- be unable to stay focused on a task or conversation
- get stuck thinking about one particular idea even when things around change or the conversation changes
- be easily distracted by things that would normally seem unimportant
- be withdrawn and not want to engage in any activity
- not respond, or seem unaware of what is happening around them.

Poor thinking skills

The person may:

- be disorientated to time and place, or person, not knowing who people are, where they are or the date
- have poor memory, particularly for recent events
- have difficulty speaking or finding the right word
- be rambling in their speech or say things which appear to be nonsense
- have trouble understanding what other people are saying
- have difficulty reading or writing.

Changes in behaviour

The person may:

- experience hallucinations, hearing or seeing things that are not there
- be restlessness, agitated or walk about with a distressed expression
- behave in a way that appears to be aggressive
- call out, moan or make other sounds
- be slower in the movements or actions or appear sleepier
- have disturbed sleep, being more awake at night and asleep during the day.

Emotional disturbance

The person may experience:

- anxiety or fear
- paranoia, believing that people are trying to harm them or others, for example that someone is trying to poison them
- depression
- irritability or anger
- euphoria, feeling excited or very happy
- apathy, a lack of interest inor enthusiasm for doing things
- rapid and unpredictable changes in mood
- changes in personality – a person who was very quiet can become louder or a person who was very jolly can appear quieter.

Types of delirium

There are three types of delirium.

Hyperactive delirium

Hyperactive delirium is the easiest to recognise. This is because the person is doing more and carers find the behaviour difficult to understand and don't know what to do. It can include restlessness, walking about, agitation, rapid mood changes or hallucinations.

Hypoactive delirium

This may be less likely to be detected as the person's behaviour is not presenting difficulties for carers. Hypoactive delirium can include inactivity or reduced movement, sluggishness, abnormal drowsiness or the person may seem to be in a daze. While this type of delirium may be less obvious, it still needs urgent medical treatment.

Mixed delirium

Mixed delirium includes both hyperactive and hypoactive symptoms. The person may quickly switch back and forth between hyperactive and hypoactive states.

Offering care

A delirium can be a terrifying experience for the person and very distressing for those who care for them. The hallucinations can be very vivid and are real to the person which can cause significant distress. For example, the person may believe a stranger is in the room with them and this can be very frightening for them. People often behave "out of character", which can be very difficult for families. A kind, gentle person may become aggressive and use language that other people can find offensive during an episode of delirium.

Often the person will not realise that they are unwell or will forget that they are unwell and want to go home. They may find it hard to understand why they need to receive care or take medication. The person may believe they are being imprisoned or poisoned, which can add to the distress of the person and those around them. If the person believes that others are trying to hurt them, it can make it very difficult to reassure and offer support. If the person doesn't understand what is happening they may attempt to defend themselves and behave in ways that are misinterpreted as physical and verbal aggression; for example, resisting support from a member of staff because they believe this person is attacking them, or attempting to break the windows to escape from being held hostage. An awareness that the person may be having these experiences and be frightened can help us to try to find ways to reassure them and offer support.

DEHYDRATION

Mild dehydration can cause tiredness, headache and a lack of concentration but in more severe cases, it can cause confusion and delirium.

Adults should drink between six and eight glasses of fluid each day. There are many reasons why a person with dementia may become dehydrated:

- The person may forget to take a drink or forget where they have left their drink.

- For some people, the part of the brain that sends a message to let you know that you are thirsty is not working properly, so the person does not recognise that they need to take a drink.

- Lack of mobility may prevent a person from independently getting a drink when they feel thirsty.

- Some medications can have a diuretic effect. More frequent urination means fluids are lost more quickly.

- Illness that causes diarrhoea and vomiting can lead to a loss of fluids.

- Feeling generally unwell can reduce the motivation to drink fluids.

- In the later stages of dementia, it can become harder to swallow as the part of the brain that sends messages to the mouth and throat may be damaged.

Symptoms of dehydration

- Increase in confusion or delirium.
- Urinating less than four times a day.
- Urine is dark and strong smelling and may also cause pain on urination.
- Dry skin mouth, lips and eyes.
- Urinary tract infections.
- Headache.
- Lowered blood pressure.
- Feeling thirsty.
- Feeling tired, dizzy or lightheaded.

Preventing dehydration

Offer a variety of drinks and foods that are high in fluids.

Make drinking easier by using cups that can be used independently and are within easy reach. If the person cannot drink independently, support them to drink at regular intervals throughout the day.

CONSTIPATION

Constipation is generally indicated if there are fewer than three bowel movements per week. It can prevent the bladder from emptying fully, which in turn can cause a UTI. Constipation can cause a stomach ache and the feeling of being bloated, feeling unwell, and a lack of energy and irritability.

The most common causes include:

- Not eating enough fibre, such as fruit, vegetables and cereals.
- Dehydration.
- With poor mobility, people with dementia often do not get enough exercise.

- Ignoring the urge or failing to recognise the urge to go to the toilet.
- Change in diet or daily routine.
- Stress, anxiety or depression.
- Side effect of medication.

MEDICATIONS

Many people living with dementia can be prescribed multiple medications and at times there are changes made to medications. In most cases, these medications help to maintain health and wellbeing. Any medication, however, can have adverse side effects.

Although all medications can cause side effects, a few commonly used drugs are known to increase the risk of confusion and falls in older adults. These include:

- Anticholinergic medications prescribed for a number of conditions, including overactive bladder, itching/allergy, vertigo, nausea, and some medications for nerve pain or depression.
- Sedatives and tranquilisers prescribed for sleep or for anxiety.

There can also be side effects due to a medication having a stronger effect on older people:

- Blood pressure medications at a dose that brings blood pressure down too far. This can result in lightheadedness, or even falls, when an older person stands.
- Diabetes medication that reduces blood sugar levels too much. This can cause falls and has been linked to faster cognitive decline.

Some drugs tend to interact with others so if there is a change in medication and a change in the person's behaviour or no change in their symptoms it is important to discuss this with their GP. If a person is started on a new medication, it is important to monitor if it is having an impact.

SENSORY IMPAIRMENT

Some types of dementia can cause damage to the brain which may appear to be a sight or hearing problem without an eye or ear condition causing this (see earlier section on cognition).

Many people with dementia will experience sensory impairment, for example sight loss, hearing loss or both, which is not related to their dementia. These sight and hearing difficulties can sometimes be misinterpreted as resulting from dementia. For example, if a person cannot follow a conversation it may be assumed that this is because of their dementia rather than because they cannot hear what is being said. If a person fails to recognise family or friends, this may be because of poor vision rather than dementia.

Sight and hearing loss can make life extremely difficult for a person who is already having to work harder to make sense of what is going on around them. It will also make communication more difficult. A person with dementia who has sight problems is more likely to fall and have difficulty finding their way around and recognising where they are. A person with dementia who has hearing loss is more likely to feel isolated from other people and experience depression.

If hearing and sight loss are managed well, this can help the person to cope better with their dementia. Both dementia and sensory loss can change and deteriorate. Regular hearing and sight tests are important to ensure that impairment does not make the challenges of dementia worse. Ensure glasses are clean and properly fitting, hearing aids are clean, switched on and working and both are within easy reach. The person may not recall that they wear glasses or use a hearing aid so offering support to put them on may be necessary. They may not recognise what the hearing aid is for or when they do remember to wear it, how to use it effectively. They may fiddle with it or refuse to wear it regularly. If the glasses or hearing aid appear to cause the person increased distress then they should not be used. If this happens it may be appropriate to seek advice from an optician or audiologist.

If a person with dementia is unable to communicate problems they are having with their sight or hearing, this is likely to cause distress. They may well be frustrated or aggressive, but unable to say why. Their behaviour may be interpreted as being a result of the dementia rather than their frustration with being unable to see or hear.

Dementia combined with sight loss can lead to:

- profound disorientation and isolation
- an increased risk of falls
- difficulties moving between light and dark spaces
- difficulties learning to use new equipment
- less independence
- increased anxiety and worry
- frustration
- misperception, misidentification or misinterpreting people, objects and activities they are looking at. For example, they may see a face in a patterned curtain, or see a shadow on the floor, but interpret it as a hole in the ground
- increased risk of experiencing hallucinations.

Dementia combined with hearing loss can lead to:

- isolation
- less independence
- misperception or misinterpreting of what people say
- increased anxiety and worry
- frustration.

Social isolation is one of the biggest challenges, but with some awareness, and more understanding of sight and hearing problems, staff and family carers are better placed to support people to continue to be engaged in the world around them.

LONG-TERM HEALTH CONDITIONS

As people get older there is a greater chance that they will be living with a long-term health condition. Any long-term health condition can cause the person to feel tired, weak and can make it hard to concentrate. All of these things can affect how the person feels and their behaviour.

Incontinence

Many people with dementia experience incontinence. The person can feel embarrassed, frustrated, or ashamed, and have a desire for privacy and independence. How we engage with the person during support with incontinence can either help them to feel better or increase their distress.

All of these conditions which impact on emotional and physical wellbeing can lead to aggression, restlessness, agitation or noisiness. The same behaviour can be present but for different reasons. When we understand what may be contributing to the behaviour, we can re-label the behaviour and find ways to support the person to reduce their distress.

ACTIVITY AND ENVIRONMENT
ACTIVITIES OF DAILY LIVING, PERSONAL CARE AND ENVIRONMENT

Many people with dementia move from being independent with personal care and activities of daily living to requiring support with both. This can be a challenge for a lot of people and can be more difficult if the person does not have insight into the changes in their ability and so does not understand that they need support.

Think about what you do first thing in the morning. Do you get out of bed straight away or do you like to stay in bed for a while, contemplating getting up? If you wear glasses or a hearing aid, do you usually put these on first so that you can see and hear what is going on? How does the person with dementia like to greet the day? Can you support them to start the day the way they would choose to, at a pace that suits them?

It is important to know if the person recognises that they need support because if they don't they may resist your help. If this is the case, how you approach them and how you offer the support will be very important.

Say, "Hello Andrew, I'm Joan the care worker" and give the person time to process what you have said.

Say "How are you today?", give the person time to process this and respond, and then you can hold out your hand and say, "Shall I help you to get out of bed?" If the person declines, give them time. Do they know who you are and why you are there? Remind them who you are. Engage them in conversation to help the person to feel safe.

Give them time to understand what is going on and why you are there. "I'm Joan the care worker. I'm here to help if you need me." Different ways of interacting will work for different people.

Most of us are private people and accepting support with personal care can be a very difficult experience. The person may experience an invasion of privacy – it can be embarrassing if your body is exposed and you are being washed by another person. They may also feel cold when their clothing is removed during personal care. When we get out of bed from under the duvet in the morning there can be a dramatic change in temperature and it can feel cold. Getting up and moving around warms us up. The person with dementia may be moving little and so is more likely to feel the cold and remain cold when their covers are removed in bed. Helping them to stay warm while getting washed and dressed will make the experience more comfortable and reduce potential distress. It is also important to protect the person's dignity and keep them covered as much as possible to reduce their embarrassment and distress, which will also keep them warm.

Support to use the toilet can be a difficult experience for many people. Some people without dementia do not like using public toilets and some even feel uncomfortable if other people hear them in the toilet. How would you feel if someone was in the room with you when you use the toilet? The person with dementia may be uncomfortable and embarrassed. When you use a public toilet do you squat, sit on the seat or wipe the seat before you sit down? When supporting a person with dementia to go to the toilet, do you do the same for them as you do for yourself? If not, why not? If the person resists support with using the toilet, can you think why? In many care homes there are staff toilets and resident toilets. Why? As a member of staff, would you use the resident's toilet? If not, why not? What is the difference between the staff and residents' toilets?

Many people are slow to eat their meals or needs support to eat meals. If they eat slowly, there is a chance the food may be cold before they finish it all. Would you finish your dinner if it was cold, or would you heat it up? Do you do the same for the person with dementia as you would do for yourself? Are there foods you don't like?

Do you know what foods the person you are caring for likes and dislikes? Are you offering them something that they would never eat? Part of the experience of eating is what the food looks like. Some people require a soft diet. What does the food look like? Is it appetising? Would you like to eat the food you are offering the person with dementia? What if the person was used to eating fish and chips from a takeaway on Friday? They may no longer be able to this now or tell you that's what they want.

The person may be sitting at a dining table with people they don't know and it can be noisy at times. What is the experience like and how would you feel if it was you?

Stop and think about the support offered to the person with dementia and how it might feel if you were on the receiving end of this support. What is the experience of their day? If this was you or a member of your family, is there anything you would change so that they would have a different experience?

ACTIVITY

Think about how you spend your day. You may have a job, paid or unpaid, or caring responsibilities for children or others which take up your time. You are also likely to have household responsibilities, shopping, cooking, cleaning or DIY. Most people will also engage in some form of leisure activity which they enjoy. This may be watching TV, reading, spending time with friends, getting some exercise, playing games or doing something creative. These activities are an escape from the demands of the day and a chance to relax. All of these things – work, household chores and leisure activities – give structure to your week and offer you a range and variety of things to think about and engage in. They give purpose and meaning to life. What does the week of the person with dementia look like? Do they have access to a range of things to occupy them? If not, why not? Is it because of their ability? Are there activities they could engage in that are appropriate for their level of ability?

Most people look forward to a holiday, a break from the routine, but after two weeks' holiday many people look forward to getting back to a routine and structure. At other times when things have been particularly busy, some people may just want to sit around for a weekend and do very little. This can be great but after a couple of days they feel the need to get up and do something. If you have ever been at home unwell, perhaps with a broken bone, the first few days may be ok but you get bored with being at home if you're not able to do anything. The days can seem long and you look forward to having something to do or company to break the monotony of the day.

Sometimes when people retire from work they believe that everything is going to be great. There will be no more stresses and demands of work. The reality of retirement can be very different. For some people their mood can deteriorate as they are at a loss with no role, structure or purpose to their day. They can feel quite isolated as they have less contact with others. The people who cope best with retirement are people who have a range of things to occupy their day or people to spend time with.

What if you didn't have a job, caring responsibilities, household chores or leisure activities to pursue? What would you spend your day doing? What if you had no purpose to your day, every day?

What about a person living with dementia? What purpose do they have to their day if they are no longer working, no longer have household chores to keep them busy or activities to engage in?

People living at home may still engage in some activity and household chores but as the dementia develops there is a tendency for others to start to do more for them. They start to lose responsibility for doing things they would normally have done. They may no longer be able to engage in or enjoy the leisure activities they used to.

What about a person living in a care home? Many people have little to occupy their day. There may be group activities offered in the care home. Are these the activities the person enjoyed before they had dementia, and do they still enjoy them? Are they at a stage in their dementia where they can still engage in these activities? Is there the opportunity to access individual activities that they enjoy and can still participate in? Is there enough variety in their day to stimulate them?

Purposeful, meaningful activity is important to all of us and this doesn't change with a diagnosis of dementia. People living with dementia have the same needs for activity as everyone else. The challenge is that they may need support to access this activity. They may not be able to engage in all the activities they did before they developed dementia but there are many things they can still enjoy.

How can you help?

- Try to engage the person with activities that they enjoy.

- Remember that they may need help to start an activity if their motivation is reduced because of the dementia.

- Avoid activities that are too difficult or too easy for their level of ability.

- Introduce a small amount of the activity at a time to avoid the person become distracted too easily.

- Focus more on doing the activity rather than the end result.

- Help the person to engage with and feel included in group activities or, if they don't want to take part, support them to watch if they wish to.

- Offer some activities that do not require active participation, such as listening to music or watching TV.

- Involve the person in chores where possible, such as dusting, setting the table, folding laundry.

Activity will give the person purpose and help them to feel valued and productive.

ENVIRONMENT

People who are living in their own home where they have lived for many years can have difficulty finding their way around their own house when they have dementia. In the kitchen, they can forget what cupboards things are kept in. For a person who has moved to a care home, it can be difficult to learn their way around their new home. Do they know how to get from the living room to the bathroom, for example? If someone needs to go to the toilet and can't find it or if they want to go to the quiet and privacy of their room and can't get there this will be very distressing.

Making changes to the environment can help to compensate for poor memory, vision and visuospatial difficulties:

- Put signs, arrows and pictures on doors and cupboards.

- Check that there is good lighting.

- Use contrasting colours on floors, walls and furniture. Bathroom fittings that contrast with floors and walls can help people to identify the toilet. It is also harder to find a white towel in a white bathroom compared with a blue towel.

- Mark the beginning and end of stairs and steps with different textures or colours.

- Use tablecloths and mats that contrast with crockery to help people easily see the food on their plate.

- Ensure the environment is clear and uncluttered. This will help people to find things and reduce the risk of falls.

A noisy environment can increase distress and can make communication more difficult.

- Reduce background noise from the television when appropriate.

- If the environment is noisy and a person seems to be distressed, support them to go to a quiet area.

- If a person has poor hearing, take them to a quiet area when talking to them.

- Ensure the person can see you when you are talking to them, as your body language may help them to understand.

Is there the opportunity for privacy? We all enjoy time on our own. If people are living in communal spaces, do they have opportunity during the day to spend time on their own? Some people enjoy being in the company of others and other people prefer their own company. Being with other people can be a comfort for some and for others it can cause them distress.

Changes to the environment

When we live at home we usually live with the same people every day. There are, of course, times when we have visitors. While we are usually very happy to see visitors, we are also sometimes glad when they have gone and we get the house back to normal again. When a person has dementia, there can often be changes to the pattern of visitors in their home. Carers may come in to offer support. There will usually be a number of different people who come in at different times and different days across the week. They have strangers coming into the privacy of their home and taking over their kitchen, coming into their bedroom and coming into the toilet with them. The person may get used to someone then that person leaves the job and they are allocated a different person to support them. All these changes can be very unsettling and increase the distress for the person with dementia.

There are also challenges for a person who moves into a care home. They are now living 24 hours a day, seven days a week with people they do not know and they did not choose to live with, many of whom also have dementia. Some of the residents with dementia may walk up to them and try to lift their things, they may enter their bedroom uninvited and they may be noisy at times. The environment can feel very unpredictable. It may also feel scary and unsafe.

There are also multiple members of staff who do a variety of things across different shifts in the day. The staff who are there in the morning are not the same people who are there at night. The person offering support at night is different from the person who offered support in the morning. The person offering support one morning may be different from the person offering support the next morning. The staff and residents all have different personalities and there are some people the person may get on with and some people they don't. This is normal, we don't all get on with everyone. But they have little choice in who offers them support. A person can become settled with the other residents and staff and then things can suddenly change. For example, at times there are new residents or new members of staff. The person may think, "Who are these people?" "What are they doing here?" "Where is Mrs Smith?" "When can I go home?"

If we understand that this may be how the person is feeling, it can change how we talk to them and offer them support.

Think about a typical day for the person with dementia. From they get up in the morning until they go to bed at night, or for the person who is in bed all day. What is the day like for them? What would it feel like if you had that kind of day? Is there anything that you could do differently that would change their experience and make their day better?

RELATIONSHIPS

Chapter 3 invites you to think about the things that are most important to you. Most people list a person or people as being the most important: children, spouse, parents, siblings, friends and extended family. Our relationships with other people are extremely important to us. How you interact with the person with dementia can impact on the quality of the relationship you have and the quality of their life.

What is the quality of relationships that the person with dementia has with other people? Have they been able to maintain relationships with family and friends? What about their relationships with carers? If they are in a care home, what is the quality of their relationships with staff and other residents?

The section on life story described how we all have people we enjoy talking to in social situations and other people we tend to avoid because we feel we have less in common with them. You usually find it easier to talk to people you feel you have something in common with, and they seem interested in what you are saying. If you get little feedback from a person you are talking to, you assume they aren't interested. You may feel uncomfortable and try to leave the situation as soon as you can and find someone else to talk to. You would probably avoid being in their company again if you could.

When talking to a person with dementia, it can be harder for them to understand what you are saying and respond. You may decide that they are not interested in what you are saying. Or you may assume that they have not understood what you have said. You may not have given them time to answer before you say something else or move away. It's our responsibility to change how we engage with the person because they don't have the ability to change how dementia has affected their ability to communicate and understand. If we don't do this, what does the relationship feel like to us or to the person with dementia?

Have you ever had the experience of being in company and the people around you are talking and not involving you in conversation? Even worse, you are sitting in between two people who are having a conversation across you and you are not included. It's rude and it shouldn't happen. What would it feel like if people talked to each other and ignored you and talked about you as if you weren't there? What if they were doing something to you and didn't ask your permission or your opinion?

You would feel disempowered, you might feel small, worthless or angry. These are the experiences that many people with dementia can have.

For some people with dementia it may sometimes feel as if they have disappeared. People around them talk but, because they can't communicate effectively, they are not fully included in the conversation in a way that they can participate. It is sometimes assumed that they can't understand so there is no point in trying. A person with dementia may not understand all of what is being said but they can understand if we are being friendly and respectful. Include the person in the conversation. Speak slowly in short sentences and give them time to process what has been said. Tone of voice and body language will show that they are cared for and are safe. The person will feel respected.

For many of us there have been times when we have been in the company of another person but we can't recall all the details of what was said. One example may be if we are having a disagreement with someone and it is an emotionally charged situation. While we may not remember all the details of what was said we do remember how it made us feel. The same is true for a person with dementia. They may not understand or remember all of what is said but they will remember how you made them feel. Every time we engage with a person with dementia we have the opportunity to make them feel valued and cared for.

If you don't have a connection with another human, it could be a very lonely life and days could be very long and frightening. We feel safer with people we know than with strangers. We decide whether strangers are safe by the way they treat us. It's not always what they say but it's how they say it and their body language. There are some people we get on well with and others that for some reason we get on less well with. The same is true for a person with dementia. There will be some carers to whom they respond well when offered support and others that they respond less well to. When this happens and a person is more distressed with some carers than others it may be related to the approach of the carers or the way that they engage. It can be helpful to look at how different staff do things differently. The way in which one carer engages may create a relationship in which the person feels safe where with another, the relationship may feel unsafe.

RELATIONSHIPS WITH FAMILY AND FRIENDS

Chapter 3 discusses some of the losses associated with dementia. This includes the loss of relationships. As the dementia progresses and old ways of interacting are no longer appropriate, it is usually important to find new ways to remain connected. Have family and friends been able to find ways to remain connected or has dementia impacted on some of these very important relationships? There may be a change in the relationship but it can still be a good quality relationship.

There are many reasons why relationships decline as dementia progresses. People have busy lives and many commitments which means that visiting is not always possible. The person may no longer be able to communicate on the phone, by email, letter, text, or by other means.

It can be distressing for family to see their loved one change with dementia, and they want to remember them as they were. The person may not recognise their family, which can be distressing. The person may become distressed when the family leave. All of these things can make visiting harder. While this can be distressing for family, what must it be like for the person to lose all those who are dear to them?

Even if your mother/father/husband/wife doesn't recognise who you are, they can recognise kindness, warmth and love. Spending time with them, reminiscing with photographs, will help them to feel safe and you can remain connected as someone who loves them, even if they don't remember what your relationship is.

Activity can be essential to help maintain relationships. An activity can be used during a visit to help you to engage with and connect with the person. This can be particularly important for people who find it difficult to communicate.

Most of us have family or friends, people we love, who have moved away from us. We don't see them as often as we used to or as we want to but we don't forget them. We think about them, talk about them, look at photos and reminisce. All of these things keep them in our mind and can help us to cope with the separation. People with dementia are no different. They will miss the important people in their life, their family and friends, when they don't see them. Talking about them or looking at pictures can help them reminisce and keep their family in their mind, even if they don't see them in person.

CARE RELATIONSHIPS

If you didn't know the person with dementia before they developed dementia, it's harder to know how best to engage with them. What do you talk about? If you talk, do they even understand what you are saying? How do you develop a relationship? This is why their life story is so important (see earlier section on life story). It opens up opportunities for connection.

If you are providing care to the person with dementia, what is your relationship like? Is it a warm relationship where the person feels safe or is it solely a task-focused relationship where you support the person to get washed, dressed, use the toilet or eat? Does the person feel as if you care for them as a person or do they feel that you are doing your job? If you were receiving support the way the person with dementia is, how would you feel?

Does the person with dementia have social interactions with carers or staff throughout the day just to spend time chatting or engaging in an activity? Or do carers and staff only engage with the person when they have to support them with their physical care need? What would the world be like if people only spoke to you when they had to support you to do something? Are the person's psychological care needs for social interaction and purposeful activity being met as well as their physical care needs?

A care relationship is a very valuable relationship and for some people with dementia these are the only relationships they have left, which makes them even more important. The way care and support are offered can have a profound impact on the quality of life of the person with dementia. It doesn't have to take more time. We just need to remember that they are a valuable person with a life lived, the same as us.

RELATIONSHIPS WITH OTHER RESIDENTS

Does the person with dementia engage with other residents in the care home? Do they have anything in common with the other residents? Is the stage of their dementia earlier or more progressed than the other residents? People with young onset dementia, those who are more active and those who are at an earlier stage in their dementia can find adjusting to life in a care home more difficult. If they feel they are different from the other residents they can feel isolated and may identify more with staff. The person may seek to spend more time with staff and staff may misinterpret this as attention seeking when in fact the person is looking for company and trying to make sense of their situation. If staff do not recognise this they can find the behaviour difficult to understand and may not know what to do.

It is possible that the person may not understand what other residents are saying or their behaviour at times. What would it feel like living in a care home with strangers that you do not know who, at times, can be unpredictable? What would it be like if you spent your days, every day with people you don't know or have little in common with?

SAFETY IN RELATIONSHIPS

Chapter 7 discusses the importance of safety. Physical safety is important but also psychological safety. We feel safe and secure in the relationships we value. Does the person with dementia have relationships that they feel safe in and secure with?

Most people don't live their lives alone, they seek company and safety. When we socialise, we socialise with people. When you go to a party, you go with people you know or you look for people you know as soon as you get there. They are your safe base at the party. You know you won't be on your own. For the person with dementia, do they have a safe base, do they know they are not alone?

Chapter 9

THE EXPERIENCE OF CARERS

UNDERSTANDING CARERS

The experience of caring for a person with dementia is different for everyone, in part because every person with dementia is different but also because every carer is different. It will depend on the type of dementia, the stage of dementia, the support available, the relationship, the unique history of the person with dementia, and the unique history of the carer. The experience of carers can also be different if they are family and friends rather than paid carers.

Whatever the situation, caring for someone with dementia means that you are likely to have to make changes to how you do things to meet the needs of the person. As the person's needs change you may have to make further changes to how you do things. Caring requires resilience, flexibility and creativity as well as patience, understanding, empathy and many more qualities.

Carers can experience a number of pressures and stresses throughout their day in addition to the many rewarding experiences of caring. There are multiple demands placed on their time and there can be moments throughout the day when they can be very busy or experience increased stress.

THE EXPERIENCE OF FAMILY AND FRIENDS WHO ARE CARERS

Dementia can feel like a bereavement, but the person is still alive. They are physically there but the emotional and psychological relationship changes as the dementia progresses.

Carers don't often recognise and reflect on the losses they are experiencing. The grief that is associated with these losses may not be recognised as grief. The focus is often on the person with dementia and their needs. People don't normally think about grieving for a person who is still alive. With dementia, there is a psychological loss before the physical loss.

Sometimes it can feel like a rollercoaster. Some days are better than others or some days the person may appear to be more like they used to be and on other days the person changes again. At times, the carer can feel as if they are just getting to understand how to manage and then things change. There can be a feeling of uncertainty, not knowing how the dementia is going to develop or what is going to change next. This may not be the experience for everyone, but it is for many people. How do you cope with a changing situation with no certainty about what the future holds? It may feel overwhelming at times.

With most terminal medical conditions, there is an opportunity to share feelings about the illness and resolve any conflicts. With dementia, there is limited opportunity to do this because of changes in thinking, reasoning and communication. This can lead to feelings of regret that remain unresolved.

Experiencing conflicted emotions is a normal reaction to an abnormal loss. The carer wants the person to continue living but, at times, they want the pain to be over. They are accepting and happy that the person is still there but at the same time grieving what has been lost.

Changes in personality and loss of shared personal memories may mean that the person with dementia does not appear to be the same person, but yet they are. The psychological connection has changed. The relationship is no longer balanced, one person depends on the other. The challenge is to maintain the bonds and connections and develop new ways of interacting.

To adapt to this new life requires the carer to take on new responsibilities and learn a different way of communicating. Family and friends may have a long history with the person and during this time have developed ways of interacting. Some of these may be helpful and some unhelpful. Some of these may need to change when a person has dementia. This can be very difficult and it is the family and friends who have to change how they interact as the person with dementia is very unlikely to be able to change. This can be more difficult if there is a history of poor relationships.

Carers also need to take care of their own needs. There are high rates of anxiety and depression in family carers (Mahoney *et al.* 2005). If the carer becomes unwell they will be unable to continue to care.

Spend a few minutes thinking about your retirement and what you plan to do?

When you think about your retirement, most people look forward to having time to do the things they have not had time to do when they were working. We work hard throughout our lives, look after our children and look forward to a long and happy retirement. We may have plans and dreams about what it will be like when we retire. When you think about what you are going to do, it is usually with someone. We plan to spend our retirement in the company of family and friends. Then things change and one half of the partnership develops dementia. What now, what about all the plans we made? The long and happy retirement has been stolen. We didn't plan to be caring for our spouse, which means we have to adapt our plans. We love the person so we will happily do it but we have experienced a loss – the loss of the planned future – and there is a need to plan a different future.

The transition from being a husband/wife to a carer is not always an easy one. There may be times when you think:

"This is not what I signed up for."

"It wasn't part of the plan to be the carer for my husband/wife."

"When I said for better or worse I wasn't thinking about dementia."

Then you might experience guilt for having these thoughts. This is a normal experience. Dementia is not something people wish for and it's normal to feel angry, frustrated and wish that the person did not have dementia.

Your best friend, the one you discussed plans and worries with, is no longer available to do this in the same way. You used to make joint decisions and now you are faced with making the decisions on your own. Where is your quality time? You don't want to look after your husband/wife, you want to be enjoying your lives together. This is what it can be like some days. Other days it can be easier and you are resigned to your role of carer and filled with love for the person you married. They are still there and you still love them. This doesn't mean it's not lonely sometimes.

How does it feel if the person no longer seems like your husband because they don't recognise you or engage with you the way your husband did but they still are your husband? A person who was normally quiet is now more talkative or a person who was very jolly is now withdrawn. Who is this person I am living with? This is not my husband/wife. I miss the person I married. You still love your husband but you may not feel love for the way the person now engages with you. The same is true if it is your wife. How do you manage the conflict of these feelings? It may feel like a separation from the person with dementia, a separation from the life once lived and the anticipated future together.

Acknowledging the loss, tolerating the range of difficult emotions and finding ways to adapt to this new life helps people to cope. Loss – reflecting on what you had before and what you had planned for the future. Frustration – why are they doing this? Guilt – sometimes I don't like them, sometimes I have said things that I don't mean. Exhaustion – I can't do this anymore. The relationship has changed and you need to find a new way to connect to maintain your relationship.

Sometimes when someone is diagnosed with dementia the husband/wife/family feels that they can care on their own. They don't want to access support from outside the family. Everyone needs a break from caring. It is a 24-hour-day, seven-days-a-week job and it can be hard and tiring. There can sometimes be a reluctance to "air your dirty laundry", particularly in a marriage, and how can you tell strangers that you cannot care for your own husband/wife? How can you tell strangers about some of the things that your husband/wife does now that are very uncharacteristic?

FRED

Fred, who has vascular dementia, came downstairs every morning, went into the living room and went behind the curtain. This caused his wife, Sadie, a lot of distress. Why is my husband, a grown man, "hiding" behind the curtain? What will the neighbours think? Fred was not showing any signs of distress while he was behind the curtain. Sadie spent over 15 minutes each morning trying to get him to come out. As she persisted, showed her frustration and raised her voice, Fred started to become distressed.

It wasn't clear why he did this but it was something that he wanted or needed to do. It may have been that when he was a young child this was a game he enjoyed playing with his parents. There were no family members who were able to provide this information. In some ways, it didn't really matter why he did it, as long as it was not causing him distress or presenting any risk to him or to others. Fred didn't think he was doing anything wrong but Sadie was annoyed with him. Was he actually doing anything wrong?

Fred and Sadie were both distressed each morning but Fred's distress was caused by Sadie's interpretation and reaction to his behaviour. Fred shouldn't be hiding behind the curtain. He needs to get out of there, come into the kitchen and get his breakfast. Fred, behind the curtain, was wondering why Sadie was so cross with him. What had he done wrong?

What needed to happen? Whose behaviour needed to change? Sadie was asked to think about why she was upset with Fred going behind the curtain in the morning. He was not hurting himself or anyone else so did it matter? When Sadie stopped to think about this, it didn't really matter. The neighbours knew that Fred had dementia. They may have noticed Fred at the window and wondered what he was doing. And then what? Spending some time thinking about why it bothered her left Sadie thinking that it didn't really matter and therefore the behaviour didn't need to stop. This was quite a shift for Sadie and isn't always easy to do. What did it matter if the neighbours saw? What did it matter what the neighbours thought? What was more important, what Fred was feeling or what the neighbours may or may not be thinking?

It took some time for Sadie to adjust to this. She had to think differently about the behaviour and what it meant. This is not always easy. When you make that shift, everything changes. But the shift doesn't happen overnight. Sadie was experiencing a loss – a loss of a relationship she once had and a transition to a new relationship which she didn't choose and can't change. Sadie had to think about what was most important and compromise, and this is not an easy decision. Caring for a person with dementia requires flexibility, compromise and adapting to changes in behaviour. Remaining in traditional fixed patterns of behaviour and interaction is not always possible.

For some people, the hardest part is actually telling someone about the behaviour. Talking about it and how it affects you. When you do this, you open up possibilities for support and ways to help you cope.

Sadie tried a few things. Sadie went into the living room and said, "Where's Fred?", loud enough so that he could hear. Sometimes he would come out from behind the curtain and sometimes he wouldn't. If he didn't, she would wait five minutes, go into the living room again and say, "Fred, breakfast is ready." Again sometimes he would come out and sometimes he wouldn't. After five, minutes she would go back to the living room and go behind the curtain to Fred and say, "Fred, your toast is on the table." She wasn't cross or annoyed and her tone was friendly. Fred always came out with a smile on his face and had his breakfast.

Sadie adapted to Fred's behaviour. She had to change how she responded, which wasn't easy and required her to compromise and change her thoughts about what the behaviour meant. In time, this just became part of their routine and she didn't think about it. It didn't cause her any distress and Fred was not distressed. Some months later Fred stopped doing this. As Fred's dementia progressed, many of his behaviours changed and Sadie had to learn new ways of adapting and coping. It wasn't always easy and she did get tired, annoyed and frustrated at times. She is human after all, but she realised that getting annoyed and frustrated actually made things worse. Fred wasn't doing any of these things on purpose to annoy her. He was making sense of the world he was living in with dementia.

To live with someone with dementia you need to rewrite your normal script for behaviour. You need to be flexible and adapt to a changing landscape. It can feel at times as if you are riding a rollercoaster of highs and lows. You think you know what you are doing, then things change.

Children of a person with dementia also experience loss, as they grieve the loss of a parent who is still alive. They might think, "This is my mother/father but they are not my mother/father" or "I still love them but our relationship has changed."

They move from the cared for to the caring for. It can be hard to watch your parent who has cared for and supported you all your life change, become vulnerable and need increasingly more support. When your parent no longer appears to recognise you, you may feel the relationship is lost. The children also have to negotiate a change in their relationship and finding connection and purpose in what is there now.

THE EXPERIENCE OF PAID CARERS

Paid carers of people living at home or staff in care homes generally will not have known the person before they had dementia. They may not know what kind of person they were before, the details of the full life they lived and their unique, rich history. When you know little about the person, sometimes you may see the dementia and not the person.

If someone is aggressive it may be assumed that this is who they are and they are referred to as "an aggressive person". It's not easy caring for someone who is aggressive. It's not a positive experience. This impacts on the empathy you can feel for the person. You can't help taking it personally sometimes: "I shouldn't have to go to work every day and have someone hit me."

If you are caring for someone and they resist support each time it is offered, this impacts on how you respond to them. If you have an experience where they have resisted and you have been hurt, you will be anxious when you offer support, and possibly more distant. You will want to complete the task as quickly as possible so as not to upset the person. This is a normal reaction but as a consequence, the way you engage will have less warmth. The person will experience this and it will impact on how they respond to you. There is the potential that the person will resist more and the situation can escalate.

If you don't know what the person was like before, you will not know that they are not an aggressive person, that they are normally very gentle. When you know more about them and understand why they may be behaving in this way you will be able to interpret their behaviour as a response to the misunderstanding of the situation (see Chapters 5 and 8).

So many demands are placed on the carer's time. They have several residents to support to get out of bed, washed and dressed, to have breakfast, to take their medication and go to the toilet. There is also paperwork to be completed. Then supporting with activities, lunch, the list goes on. Carers respond to multiple requests for different types of support from a range of different people throughout the day. Each person has different needs and likes to be cared for in different ways. It's challenging to get it right all the time. With so many demands on time it can be difficult to have quality relationships with the people you are caring for. Carers want to do a good job but sometimes there are so many demands on their time that they don't have enough time to get to know the person. Having brief information about the person's life story helps (see Chapter 8).

Caring is a physically and emotionally demanding job. The role involves meeting both the physical needs of the person but also their psychological needs. It can be easy for care staff to understand what the physical needs are. It is easy to see how their job can become task focused, meeting just the physical needs. The psychological needs for love, belonging and social relationships can be a second priority. But these needs are of equal importance to the physical needs. Carers and care staff often have not had sufficient training on dementia to help them fully understand the psychological needs of the people they are caring for.

For a variety of different reasons, care homes regularly need to use agency staff, who have little opportunity to get detailed information on all the residents they will care for on a shift. This can make their job more difficult and it can also add to the distress of the person with dementia. They are being cared for by another stranger but this stranger has never met them before and doesn't know how they like to be supported. Care staff want to do a good job. It is more difficult for them if they do not fully understand the person they are working with.

CLEAR Dementia Care© provides brief information on a person for care staff to help them understand that person, what their behaviour is, why they might be behaving that way and how they can be supported to reduce potential distress. These recommendations are based on a CLEAR Dementia Care© assessment, Behaviour Record Charts and other available information (see Chapter 10). Using the domains of CLEAR Dementia Care© can help to develop better understanding of the whole person and lead to better care and a better quality of life for the person with dementia. By improving the quality of their interactions, care staff will also benefit from a better experience of delivering care.

Chapter 10

SUPPORTING CARE STAFF

The aim of CLEAR Dementia Care© is to provide accessible and simple ways to assess and understand behaviour in dementia.

CLEAR Dementia Care© offers a holistic and person-centred assessment, formulation and management plan. To fully understand the meaning of a person's behaviour, it is important to try to understand the behaviour from the perspective of that person (Kitwood 1997). We need to answer questions such as: What is a typical day like for this person? What might it feel like to have this have this type of day? It is also important to try to understand the perspective of the carer(s) of the person with dementia.

CLEAR person-centred assessment is comprehensive and holistic. The goal of the assessment is to understand the behaviour in the context of the person and their environment, and identify any unmet need(s). CLEAR assessment includes the domains of Cognition, Life story and personality, Emotional and physical wellbeing, Activity and environment, and Relationships (see Chapter 8).

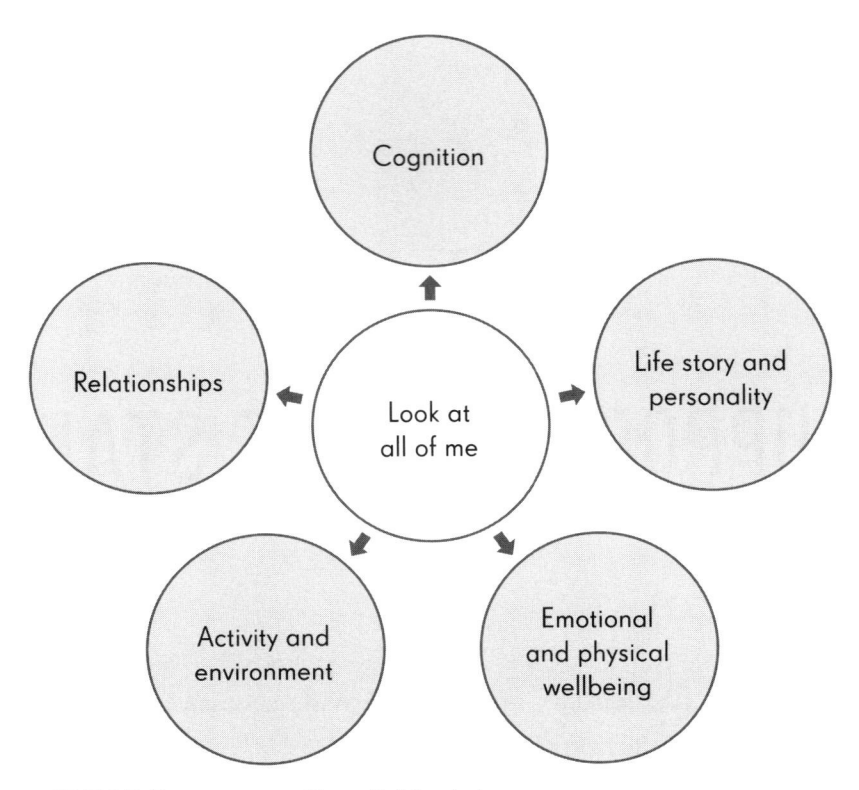

Figure 10.1: CLEAR Dementia Care© Model

© Northern Health and Social Care Trust 2018

The five CLEAR domains interact with each other and impact on behaviour. For example, a person's life story and personality prior to moving into a care home may reflect that they were someone who was very independent. Changes in cognitive function, including reduced insight, means they are unaware that they now need more support with personal care. If care staff attempt to support with personal care, the person may not understand why their support is needed or indeed what the intention of the care staff is. This will affect the relationship between the individual and the care staff, the person may resist this unwanted support and care staff may not understand why the person is refusing support. The increased dependency may have a negative impact on the person's emotional wellbeing, leading to lower self-esteem. Uncertainty about the role of the care staff may cause the person to feel anxious or scared about what is going to happen or what their intentions are. Consequently, the person may act in a way to maintain their independence or defend themselves. This, in turn, could be perceived by the care staff as aggression. We thus have two different perspectives of the behaviour. When we recognise and acknowledge the perspectives of both, we can try to find way to find ways to facilitate understanding and reduce distress.

CLEAR Dementia Care© also aims to correct unhelpful assumptions about the cause of the behaviour(s). On occasion, carers may refer to behaviour as "attention seeking". Putting the behaviour in the context of the person and their environment can dispel these unhelpful assumptions.

HELPING CARERS TO UNDERSTAND WHEN BEHAVIOURS OCCUR

Behaviour Record Charts described in Chapter 6 are used to get a sense of a "day in the life of" the person. These charts also help staff to see when specific behaviours are happening, highlight patterns in behaviour and identify strategies that may help.

Medication Record Charts are also used to record when medication is administered (Appendix 4). A review of medication is important because medication can impact on behaviour. Some medications may need to be reduced, increased, discontinued or others may need to be introduced. The Behaviour Record Charts can be reviewed in the context of the Medication Record Charts to see if there is any relationship between medication and behaviour. This can be particularly helpful when considering the impact of pain on behaviour. Looking at the pattern of administration of pain relief medication will help to identify if it has any impact on behaviour.

SHARING INFORMATION WITH CARE HOME STAFF

The long-term success of any intervention depends on successful collaboration with all of the carers of the person with dementia. The ongoing assessment and proposed management plan is discussed verbally with available staff at every review. Written feedback is also provided at every review throughout the assessment and intervention process on Initial Contact and Review documents (Duffy and Richardson, 2018). The written information is presented in a format which is accessible to all care staff. It is clear what the behaviour is, why it might be occurring and how staff should respond. It is kept as brief as possible using language that is accessible to all staff. Managers agree that all staff will read the information, and all staff are required to sign to confirm that they have read it. This facilitates ownership and commitment to the principle that it is everyone's responsibility to engage with the assessment and management process.

INITIAL CONTACT FORM

This is the summary of the behaviour(s) reported by care staff, potential causes for the behaviour(s) and recommendations of how to address any identified unmet need. For all recommendations, it is clear what needs to be done and who needs to do it. As appropriate, a member of staff is given responsibility to ensure that a given recommendation is completed. For example, at the beginning of each shift a member of staff is given the responsibility of completing the Behaviour Record Charts. Potential causes for the behaviour are based on the information gathered from the CLEAR Dementia Care© assessment. This also provides an opportunity to correct unhelpful assumptions about the cause of the behaviour(s), such as labelling behaviour "aggressive" or "attention seeking".

REVIEW OF RECOMMENDATIONS

Feedback from the ongoing assessment together with the management plan is discussed and agreed with available staff at every review. Following each review, updated written information is provided on the outcome of the assessment and management plan. This is written such that staff only have to read the most recent review to understand the behaviour and to address an identified unmet need. This is particularly important for agency staff who have not been part of the ongoing assessment process. It enables them to gain a basic understanding of the person in a short time. There is agreement that all staff sign to confirm that they have read this document.

UNDERSTANDING DOCUMENT

When all the relevant information has been gathered, a written formulation is shared with staff. The document is called Understanding [person's name]. The document is written in a way that is clear and accessible for all staff. There is agreement that all staff sign to confirm that they have read this document. This document has a number of sections.

LIFE HISTORY

Everyone has an interesting history peppered with challenges and achievements. When someone develops dementia, sometimes their history can be lost and they are seen in the context of their diagnosis, rather than the person they are. Understanding the person is a brief summary of the person's life which helps carers to see the person beyond the label of their condition. It contains enough information so that you have a better understanding of the person but it is short enough, generally no more than a half page, that all staff will have time to read it.

It is important to maintain confidentiality and therefore personal information included in this document respects confidentiality. If a person has experienced trauma, it is not appropriate to share the details of this with everyone. It may, however, be important for people to know that the person has experienced trauma if this can help explain some of their behaviours. The details of what is shared need to be considered carefully.

Assumptions about behaviour attributed to negative personality traits, for example, "the person always liked to get their own way" are not helpful and are not included in this summary. If these are included, there is a tendency to attribute the presenting behaviour to the person's personality, rather than their unmet need. The focus on strengths and achievements increases the likelihood that the perception and subsequent behaviour of the carer will change. The goal is to increase the esteem with which the person is held by those who care for them. This, in turn, positively impacts on interaction to maximise quality of life of the person with dementia.

EXPLAINING THE BEHAVIOUR

The behaviour(s) is described. Potential causes for the behaviour are based on information gathered from the comprehensive CLEAR Dementia Care© assessment. The explanation(s) is developed with staff feedback throughout the assessment process at each review. This explanation of the behaviour provides the framework for intervention strategies.

WHAT MIGHT HELP/ADDRESSING UNMET NEED

Recommendations are based on the potential causes of the behaviour(s) with clear links made between the explanation of the behaviour and the way to address the identified unmet need. Recommendations are SMART (Specific, Measurable, Achievable, Realistic and Time-scaled). They involve participation for the staff, family and friends and/or the person with dementia, as appropriate. Purposeful activity is recognised as being an essential part of daily life.

MEETING WITH CARE STAFF/CARERS

When the Understanding document has been shared with staff, a member of the team offers an informal meeting with available care staff to provide the opportunity to discuss the document and agreed plan to identify unmet needs. If appropriate, changes are made to the document.

In the Understanding document, the goal is to provide some details of the person's life story to help the care staff to get a better understanding of who the person is. When someone moves into a care home staff have little information about the life the person has led before. This information helps them to see the individual rather than a person with dementia. By the time the Understanding document is completed many of the behaviours will have reduced in frequency or resolved. Recommendations from across the reviews are included as, should the situation change and some of the behaviours re-emerge, staff will have strategies that they can try.

Chapter 11

A CASE EXAMPLE

MARGARET

Margaret is a 75-year-old lady with a diagnosis of Alzheimer's disease. She had been referred to the specialist team because staff in the care home reported that she was defecating and smearing faeces, trying to leave the care home and was verbally aggressive towards care staff.

Margaret moved into the care home four months earlier. Before this she was living at home with her husband. Margaret enjoyed walking and she and her husband would walk for three miles every day. Her husband became unwell and was no longer able to go for their daily walk. Margaret continued to want to go for a walk and had been leaving home unaccompanied. On several occasions, she was found walking around her local town unable to find her way home and very distressed. An occupational therapy assessment concluded that she was unsafe on the road when unaccompanied. There was a risk that she would attempt to cross the road without paying enough attention to whether it was safe to cross. As her dementia progressed and her husband's physical health deteriorated, he was unable to care for her safely at home. The family made the difficult decision that it was in her best interests to move into a care home.

Margaret's memory was poor. When you had a conversation with her and left the room, she did not recall the conversation. She did not recall that she was now living in a care home and did not know her way around the building. If she was in the dining room, she could not find her way back to her bedroom without support from staff. Her language and communication skills were good. If you talked with her she understood what you were saying and could respond appropriately. Her attention was fairly good and she still enjoyed looking through magazines and newspapers.

Margaret had a happy childhood. When she left school she worked in the local factory. She married David and they had four children. She stopped working to look after her children and when they were older she returned to work in a local school canteen. She was a very house-proud lady and enjoyed being a homemaker. Margaret always liked to be busy and when she retired she volunteered one day a week in a local charity shop. Margaret enjoyed holidays with her husband and they both liked being physically active. She was a private person, enjoyed the company of her family and had a few close friends. She had two brothers and two sisters with whom she was very close. Her two brothers died in the past four years. One of her sons lost part of his arm in an accident at work. Margaret was very distressed by this and often talked about what he experienced, wishing she could have taken his pain upon herself, but she also talked about how proud she was of the way he adjusted to his injury. She enjoyed spending time with her eight grandchildren. She was a great seamstress and often made dresses for her granddaughters.

Physically, Margaret was in good health. There was no evidence of pain, infection or other physical conditions that caused her discomfort or added to her confusion. There was evidence that her mood was low, her appetite was poor and she spent much of her time isolated in her room. She appeared anxious and wary of the other residents.

Margaret had little to occupy her time and she had lost access to the activities that she enjoyed. There were a number of group activities offered in the care home but Margaret declined to engage in any of these. At times, staff encouraged her to sit in the communal lounge but when she had been there for a short time she asked staff to take her back to her room. There was a garden in the care home and Margaret enjoyed being in the garden but she was unable to access the garden independently. When time permitted, staff would accompany Margaret to the garden but this did not happen regularly.

Margaret had not developed any relationships with other residents in the care home, nor had she developed relationships with staff. Her husband, David, lived a 30-minute drive from the care home as did one of her daughters, Marie. Her son,

Jack, lived a two-hour drive away and her other two daughters, Emma and Beth, lived in other countries. David tried to visit every day but, because of his ill physical health he had been unable to visit for two weeks. When Margaret first moved into the care home, Marie visited every two days. She worked and had young children and, although she tried to visit as often as possible, with her other responsibilities she came one night per week and on a Saturday afternoon. Jack visited once a month and Emma and Beth returned home one or two times each year. They had both visited on one occasion since Margaret had been in the care home. She had two close friends who visited her weekly and her grandchildren visited regularly. Margaret enjoyed seeing family and friends but they were unable to visit as often as they or Margaret would like. At times, Margaret could be very tearful when they were leaving and after they had left.

With all this information we can begin to form an impression of Margaret. She was living in a place where she did not know people and this appeared to be making her anxious. She missed her family and friends and she appeared to have little to occupy her time. She may have been finding this particularly difficult as she was someone who always liked to be busy.

How do we understand the faecal smearing, attempts to exit the building and aggression reported by staff? One way to do this is to record when these behaviours happen to see if there are any patterns. Staff were asked to complete CLEAR Dementia Care© Behaviour Record Charts. This method of recording behaviour does not require the person recording the behaviour to interpret it. They can be completed very quickly by any member of staff. At the beginning of each shift a member of staff is given responsibility for ensuring that the charts are completed. This person does not have to complete the chart for the shift but just make sure that at all times someone on the shift has responsibility for completing the chart. This requires a member of staff to have the chart and a pen in their pocket.

Staff reported that the behaviours that were causing distress for both Margaret and staff were the faecal smearing, pacing and trying to exit the building, and aggression. Staff agreed the codes that they would use for each of these behaviours: F – faecal smearing, A – aggression and P – pacing. It was also important to record when Margaret was content – C and sleeping – S. It was agreed that staff would be asked to record these behaviours for one week. This chart is shown in Figure 11.1. Recording the behaviour simply requires writing the code (F, A, C, P or S) in the chart. Margaret's chart was divided into one-hour time intervals for each day of one week.

A CLEAR Dementia Care© Initial Contact form was completed which explained the Behaviour Record Charts and why they were being used. This was to ensure that all staff were aware of what they had to do and why.

CLEAR Dementia Care© CONFIDENTIAL CDC-BRC
CLEAR Dementia Care **BEHAVIOUR RECORD CHART**
Name: **Margaret** DOB:

Time	MON	TUE	WED	THUR	FRI	SAT	SUN
8–9am							
9–10am							
10–11am							
11–12am							
12–1pm							
1–2pm							
2–3pm							
3–4pm							
4–5pm							
5–6pm							
6–7pm							
7–8pm							
8–9pm							
9–10pm							
10–11pm							
11–12pm							
12–1am							
1–2am							
2–3am							
3–4am							
4–5am							
5–6am							
6–7am							
7–8am							

Code: C – Content S – Sleeping A – Aggression P – Pacing F – Faecal smearing

Figure 11.1 Margaret's Behaviour Record Chart
© CLEAR Dementia Care & Northern Health and Social Care Trust 2018

A CASE EXAMPLE

At the end of one week, Figure 11.2 shows what Margaret's chart looked like. Highlighter pens were then used to colour code a particular behaviour. Faecal smearing is pink, aggression is red, pacing is dark blue, content is green and sleeping is light blue (see Figure 11.3).Colour coding enables us to identify any patterns in Margaret's behaviour.

CLEAR Dementia Care© CONFIDENTIAL CDC-BRC
CLEAR Dementia Care **BEHAVIOUR RECORD CHART**
Name: **Margaret** DOB:

Time	MON	TUE	WED	THUR	FRI	SAT	SUN
8–9am	A	A	A	A	A	C	A
9–10am	C	C	C	C	C	C	A
10–11am	C	C	C	P	C	C	P A
11–12am	P	C	C	F A	C	C	P A
12–1pm	C	C P	C	P	P	C P	C P
1–2pm	P	F A	P	P	F A	F A	P A
2–3pm	F A	P	F A	C	P	P	C
3–4pm	P	C	P	C	C	P	C
4–5pm	P	C	P	P	P	P	P A
5–6pm	C P	C P	C P	C P	C P	C P	C P
6–7pm	P	P	P	P	P	P	P
7–8pm	P	P	P	P	P	P	P
8–9pm	C	C	C	C	C	C	C
9–10pm	C A	C A	C	C A	C A	C	C A
10–11pm	C	C	S	C	C	S	C
11–12pm	S	S	S	S	S	S	S
12–1am	S	S	S	S	S	S	S
1–2am	S	S	S	S	S	S	S
2–3am	S	S	S	S	S	S	S
3–4am	A	S	A	S	S	S	S
4–5am	S	S	S	S	S	S	S
5–6am	S	S	S	S	S	A	S
6–7am	S	S	S	S	C	C	S
7–8am	C	C	C	C	C	C	C

Code: C – Content S – Sleeping A – Aggression P – Pacing F – Faecal smearing

Figure 11.2: Margaret's Behaviour Record Chart after one week

© CLEAR Dementia Care & Northern Health and Social Care Trust 2018

CLEAR Dementia Care©
CLEAR Dementia Care

CONFIDENTIAL
BEHAVIOUR RECORD CHART
Name: **Margaret**

CDC-BRC

DOB:

Time	MON	TUE	WED	THUR	FRI	SAT	SUN
8–9am	A	A	A	A	A	C	A
9–10am	C	C	C	C	C	C	A
10–11am	C	C	C	P	C	C	P A
11–12am	P	C	C	F A	C	C	P A
12–1pm	C	C P	C	P	P	C P	C P
1–2pm	P	F A	P	P	F A	F A	P A
2–3pm	F A	P	F A	C	P	P	C
3–4pm	P	C	P	C	C	P	C
4–5pm	P	C	P	P	P	P	P A
5–6pm	C P	C P	C P	C P	C P	C P	C P
6–7pm	P	P	P	P	P	P	P
7–8pm	P	P	P	P	P	P	P
8–9pm	C	C	C	C	C	C	C
9–10pm	C A	C A	C	C A	C A	C	C A
10–11pm	C	C	S	C	C	S	C
11–12pm	S	S	S	S	S	S	S
12–1am	S	S	S	S	S	S	S
1–2am	S	S	S	S	S	S	S
2–3am	S	S	S	S	S	S	S
3–4am	A	S	A	S	S	S	S
4–5am	S	S	S	S	S	S	S
5–6am	S	S	S	S	S	A	S
6–7am	S	S	S	S	C	C	S
7–8am	C	C	C	C	C	C	C

Code: C – Content S – Sleeping A – Aggression P – Pacing F – Faecal smearing

Figure 11.3: Margaret's Behaviour Record Chart with colour coding

© CLEAR Dementia Care & Northern Health and Social Care Trust 2018

There were discussions with staff to help understand what was going on in the care home at the time of the behaviours that might explain why the behaviours were happening. This process is very empowering for staff because they can usually provide most of the answers. It's no longer an expert team coming up with the answers but the staff themselves who spend most time with the person.

Sometimes the charts highlight that a behaviour that staff thought was happening often is not happening very frequently. It may be that other behaviours are happening more frequently. If this is the case, it may be necessary to record a different set of behaviours for one week.

For Margaret, the chart indicated that staff found her behaviour aggressive in the morning and evening when they offered support with personal care and also when they supported her following an episode of faecal smearing. Because of Margaret's dementia, she did not know who staff were when they went into her room in the morning. Margaret interpreted this as strangers invading her personal space and privacy. While Margaret was still quite independent, she needed prompting to wash and change her clothing in the morning. Her dementia also caused her some problems with sequencing, which meant that she got confused about what order to put her clothes on. When staff tried to support her with this she resisted, as she didn't have the insight to know that she needed their help and she didn't want their help. The more staff tried to help, the more distressed Margaret became.

What would help Margaret? First, it was recommended that when staff went into Margaret's room to support her with personal care they said hello and told her who they were:

- "Hello Margaret, my name is Clare, I'm a care assistant." Staff then needed to give Margaret time to respond and answer any questions she had.

- They should ask her, "Shall I help you to choose what you want to wear today?" Specific advice could be given for each step. The language used is important – it is supportive but empowering. This message is, you can do this yourself but I'm happy to help you. Margaret should be supported to be as independent as possible with each of the steps of getting washed and dressed.

It was important to talk about each of the steps one at a time, giving Margaret as much control and independence as possible with each step. This had the benefit of maintaining Margaret's skills and also maintaining her confidence that she was still able to be independent. Staff spending a little extra time with Margaret explaining who they are would help her to feel safe in the interaction. Their tone and body language would reinforce that they were safe and supportive. If all staff engaged with Margaret in the same way each morning, the morning routine would become more predictable, which would help Margaret to feel safe and secure.

When we look at Margaret's chart we can see that there was no aggression reported on Saturday morning. Staff advised that the member of staff who supported Margaret on Saturday never reported any aggression from her. It is important to know why this member of staff was different. We all have different ways of interacting. We get on with some people better than others. It is possible that Margaret got on better with that particular member of staff . It would be good to know whether this was just because of their personality or something about the way she engaged with Margaret. There may be an opportunity to learn how Margaret liked to be offered support. Was there a way that this member of staff interacted with Margaret that reduced her distress during support with personal care?

Staff advised that, after support with personal care, Margaret was supported to go to the dining room for breakfast. They reported that she did eat her breakfast, although she didn't eat very much and after breakfast she asked to go back to her room. Staff encouraged Margaret to sit in the lounge with other residents after breakfast but she usually declined and preferred to go back to her room.

At lunchtime, staff supported Margaret to the dining room and after lunch supported her to sit in a quiet area of the care home. The charts highlight that Margaret tended to pace the corridors in the early afternoon. This was a time when the care home was busier with visitors. This might have been unsettling for Margaret and she may have wanted to remove herself from the busier environment. On the Thursday, Friday and Sunday she had visitors and was more settled.

A CASE EXAMPLE

After dinner and in the early evening Margaret also tended to pace the corridors. The care home was quieter in the evening and many of the residents were in the lounge and the TV was on. Margaret did not enjoy watching TV and the impression was that she was bored in the evenings and was looking for something to do. She didn't have anything to occupy her.

The charts show that staff reported verbal aggression on Sunday morning. Staff reported that there was a church service on Sunday morning and an unusual amount of activity in the home as residents moved about to get to the service. Also, some of the resident's families attended. This may have been unsettling for Margaret and increased her anxiety. Her anxiety caused her to be sharp with staff in her tone.

There were discussions with staff about activities that Margaret could engage in. Suggested activities were folding laundry, setting the dining tables for meals and dusting the rails around the care home. Other activities were looking at magazines, newspapers and photograph albums which her daughter had agreed to bring to the care home.

Episodes of faecal smearing were reported most days, usually in the early afternoon. An observation was scheduled. After lunch, Margaret was supported by staff to sit in a quiet area of the lounge. Margaret sat in the lounge for a period of time and was observed to leave the lounge and walk along the corridor; she looked around her and went into the rooms of two other residents who asked her to leave. A member of staff approached Margaret and she asked to go to her room. She went directly to the toilet in her room and was there for some time. It appeared that Margaret had been looking for the toilet and when she couldn't find it, she had a bowel movement before she made it to the toilet. Margaret, who was a very private lady, had tried to clean herself. She had some difficulty with this and some of the faeces got onto the wall, the toilet seat and the sink. What appeared to be faecal smearing was actually Margaret's attempt to clean herself. This was discussed with staff who agreed to change the signage in the care home. It became clear that Margaret regularly had a bowel movement in the afternoon. Staff were asked to pay attention to Margaret when she left the lounge in the afternoon and if she started walking, staff were to approach her and ask if she wanted them to walk with her to her room.

Over the course of the next few weeks staff tried offering a range of activities to Margaret and she really enjoyed helping staff. As she was doing the activity she talked more to staff and this helped her to build better relationships with them. It was also agreed that Margaret would be supported to go for a walk during the day, weather permitting. Some days this was with staff and some days with friends. There was a schedule agreed for different activities which included who would be accompanying Margaret on a walk on specific days. Margaret became more settled in the care home, with a predictable routine which kept her busy. She also started to engage more in group activities in the home.

Figure 11.4 shows Margaret's chart six weeks later. There were no reported incidents of aggression. Margaret was becoming more familiar with her environment. The increased activity was helping her to build relationships with staff. Staff had changed their approach with Margaret during support with personal care. She was supported to be more independent. There had only been one incident when she was cross with a staff member during support with personal care. Margaret was participating in a number of different activities which occupied her and gave her purpose throughout the day. Staff were supporting Margaret to her room, if necessary to use the toilet, and there had been no incidents of faecal smearing reported.

A CASE EXAMPLE

CLEAR Dementia Care© CONFIDENTIAL CDC-BRC
CLEAR Dementia Care **BEHAVIOUR RECORD CHART**
  Name: **Margaret** DOB:

Time	MON	TUE	WED	THUR	FRI	SAT	SUN
8–9am	C	C	C	A	C	C	C
9–10am	C	C	C	C	C	C	C
10–11am	C	C	C	P	C	C	C
11–12am	P	C	C	C	C	C	C
12–1pm	C	P	C	C	P	C	C P
1–2pm	P	C	P	P	C	C	C
2–3pm	C	P	C	C	P	C	C
3–4pm	P	C	C	C	C	P	C
4–5pm	C	C	P	P	C	C	P
5–6pm	C P	C	C	C	C	C	C
6–7pm	C	P	C	C	P	C	P
7–8pm	P	C	P	P	C	P	C
8–9pm	C	C	C	C	C	C	C
9–10pm	C	C	C	C	C	C	C
10–11pm	C	C	S	C	C	S	C
11–12pm	S	S	S	S	S	S	S
12–1am	S	S	S	S	S	S	S
1–2am	S	S	S	S	S	S	S
2–3am	S	S	S	S	S	S	S
3–4am	S	S	S	S	S	S	S
4–5am	S	S	S	S	S	S	S
5–6am	S	S	S	S	S	S	S
6–7am	S	S	S	S	C	C	S
7–8am	C	C	C	C	C	C	C

Code: C – Content S – Sleeping A – Aggression P – Pacing F – Faecal smearing

© CLEAR Dementia Care & Northern Health and Social Care Trust 2018

Figure 11.3: Margaret's Behaviour Record Chart with colour coding

Margaret was spending more time in the lounge and enjoyed sitting with another female resident. They didn't engage in very much conversation but they appeared to be content in each other's company. Margaret enjoyed getting out for walks. Her mobility had declined so she was content to go for a short walk. She still walked the corridor frequently but staff's impression was that sometimes she was happy doing this and she enjoyed the exercise. Staff offered Margaret opportuninties to participate in an activity when she was observed to be walking the corridor. Sometimes she agreed and at other times she wanted to walk. Staff no longer saw this behaviour as a problem and Margaret did not appear to be distressed.

Information from the domains of CLEAR Dementia Care© and the Behaviour Record Charts have helped to give a better understanding of Margaret and her behaviour. Understanding her behaviour from her perspective, in the context of her day, helped staff to come up with a range of ways to support Margaret. The outcome was a reduction in her distress and an improvement in her quality of life.

CLEAR Dementia Care© helps carers to see the world from the perspective of the person with dementia. When we see the whole person and understand their perspective, we can find ways to reduce distress. The outcome is better care and enhanced quality of life.

APPENDICES

The following appendices can be downloaded at www.jkp.com/voucher using the code KAEGYFO

APPENDIX 1: BEHAVIOUR RECORD CHART

CLEAR Dementia Care© CONFIDENTIAL BRC – CDC
CLEAR Dementia Care **BEHAVIOUR RECORD CHART**
Name:_____ DOB:

Time	MON	TUE	WED	THUR	FRI	SAT	SUN
8–9am							
9–10am							
10–11am							
11–12am							
12–1pm							
1–2pm							
2–3pm							
3–4pm							
4–5pm							
5–6pm							
6–7pm							
7–8pm							
8–9pm							
9–10pm							
10–11pm							
11–12pm							
12–1am							
1–2am							
2–3am							
3–4am							
4–5am							
5–6am							
6–7am							
7–8am							

Code:

APPENDIX 2: AIDE MEMOIRE TO HELP UNDERSTAND BEHAVIOUR

CLEAR Dementia Care©   CONFIDENTIAL   AM – CDC
CLEAR Dementia Care   **AIDE MEMOIRE TO HELP UNDERSTAND BEHAVIOUR**

Below are areas which can impact on a person's behaviour. It is important to consider these as part of a comprehensive assessment.

1. Cognition	
Orientation	Does the person know where they are living and why they are in a care home? Do they know the date and time? Can they navigate around the building?
Attention	Can the person attend in conversation? Can they attend to reading, television or activities offered in the care home?
Language/ Communincation	Can the person understand verbal or written language? Can they use language to communicate? If not how do they communicate their needs? Could they use pictures to help with communication?
Memory	What can the person remember about what is said in conversation? Can they remember things that were said or happened recently (short-term memory)? Can they remember things that happened a long time ago (long-term memory)?
Visuospatial processing	Can they find their way around the building? Can they locate the food on their plate? When they reach for something are they accurate? Can they locate their clothing and co-ordinate all the movements needed to get dressed?
Delusions	Does the person have difficulty distinguishing what is real from what is imagined? Do they believe that something is true that is not true?
Hallucinations	Does the person see or hear things that other people cannot see or hear? If yes, does this cause distress?

2. Life story and personality	
Previous occupations	Brief history, including family and pervious occupations. Details of challenges and achievements.
Roles within the family	What were the person's roles within the family? What roles do they have now?
Personality	How would the person or others describe their personality prior to the onset of dementia? Has their personality changed?
Normal routines	What was their normal routine before they came into the care home? How are things different now?

cont.

© CLEAR DEMENTIA CARE & NORTHERN HEALTH AND SOCIAL CARE TRUST 2018

2. Life story and personality

Hobbies/Interests	How did they spend leisure time before coming into the care home? Do they still have the ability to engage in these activities now? Do they have the opportunity to participate in these activities now?
Likes and dislikes	What are their likes and dislikes? Are people who interact with them aware of these?

3. Emotional and physical wellbeing

Physical health	Long-term conditions and recent changes to physical health.
Infection	Has presence of infection been investigated and treated if appropriate?
Pain	Are there physical health conditions which would suggests the person is likely to experience pain? Look at CLEAR Dementia Care© Pain Checklist.
Constipation	Does the person have regular bowel movements?
Dehydration	Is the person drinking enough fluids?
Medication	Have there been recent changes in medication? Is the person taking their medication? If analgesic medication is prescribed, is it being administered, in particular is it given as needed? Side effects of medication?
Mood	If history of low mood, how did the person cope in the past? Present changes in mood? Are there issues of adjustment to recent change in environment, bereavement, loss of role, independence, activity etc? Isolated in room, change in appetite, sleep?
Anxiety	If there is a history of anxiety, how did the person cope in the past? New presentation, precipitating factors? Present situations where the person appears wary or frightened.
Other mental health	Trauma history?

4. Activity and environment

Personal care and activities of daily living	Is the person independent in personal care and activities of daily living? How much support do they need with personal care? How much support do they need with activities of daily living? Do they get enough/too much support?
Typical day	What does the person do in a typical day from when they get up until they go to bed? How often do they engage with others, change their environment or engage in activity? Is this how the person would have spent their day before coming into care? How is this different?
Participation in activities	Are there activities offered? Does the person engage in activities? Are the activities appropriate to the stage of their dementia?

Changes in environment	Have there been recent changes to the environment in which they live?
Noise	Is the environment too noisy or too quiet?
Overcrowding	How many other residents share the communal space?
Privacy	Is there opportunity for privacy?
Signage	Is it clear how to navigate around the environment and find your room/bathroom/lounge/dining room? Can they follow the signage?

5. Relationships

Relationships with family	Do family visit? Does the person have meaningful interaction with family? Have there been recent changes to the pattern of visits or any recent bereavements?
Relationships with residents	Does the person engage with other residents? Do other residents have similar levels of ability? Is the person more or less able than other residents?
Relationships with staff	How does the person engage with staff? Is there sufficient time for staff to engage in activities outside personal care?
Does the person feel safe and secure?	Is the person attempting to leave the building? Do they say they want to leave/move somewhere else? Do they appear frightened in particular rooms or at particular times?

APPENDIX 3: DOMAINS CHECKLIST

CLEAR Dementia Care© CONFIDENTIAL DLC – CDC
CLEAR Dementia Care **DOMAINS CHECKLIST**

Service user details
Name   Address   DOB

Below are areas which can impact on a person's behaviour. It is important to consider these as part of a comprehensive assessment.

1. Cognition	Comments
Orientation	
Attention	
Language/Communication	
Memory	
Visuospatial processing	
Delusions	
Hallucinations	

2. Life story and personality	Comments
Previous occupations	
Roles within the family	
Personality	
Normal routines	
Hobbies/Interests	
Likes and dislikes	

3. Emotional and physical wellbeing	Comments
Physical health	
Infection	
Pain	
Constipation	
Dehydration	
Medication	
Mood	
Anxiety	
Other mental health	

4. Activity and environment	Comments
Personal care and activities of daily living	
Typical day	
Participation in activities	
Changes in environment	
Noise	
Overcrowding	
Privacy	
Signage	

5. Relationships	Comments
Relationships with family	
Relationships with residents	
Relationships with staff	
Does the person feel safe and secure?	

Completed by
Name Designation
Signature Date

APPENDIX 4: MEDICATION RECORD

CLEAR Dementia Care©
CLEAR Dementia Care
Service user details
Name
Medications:

CONFIDENTIAL
MEDICATION RECORD

Address

MRC – CDC

DOB

Date/Time	10.00	14.00	18.00	22.00	Other
1st					
2nd					
3rd					
4th					
5th					
6th					
7th					
8th					
9th					
10th					
11th					
12th					
13th					
14th					
15th					
16th					
17th					
18th					
19th					
20th					
21st					
22nd					
23rd					
24th					
25th					
26th					
27th					
28th					
29th					
30th					
31st					

REFERENCES

Alzheimer's Research UK (n.d.) Attitutes to Dementia. Available at www.dementiastatistics.org/statistics/attitudes-to-dementia

Atkinson, R. C. and Shiffrin, R. M. (1968) "Human Memory: A Proposed System and its Control Processes." In K. W. Spence and J. T. Spence, *The Psychology of Learning and Motivation* (Volume 2), pp. 89–195. New York, NY: Academic Press.

Duffy, F. (2016) "'Look at all of me' A Clear model for dementia care." *The Journal of Dementia Care*, 22(3), 27–30.

Duffy, F. and Richardson, J. (2018) *CLEAR Dementia Care©: Handbook on Implementation with Case Presentations.* Antrim: Northern Health and Social Care Trust.

James, I. A. (2011) *Understanding Behaviour in Dementia that Challenges: A Guide to Assessment and Treatment.* London: Jessica Kingsley Publishers.

Kitwood, T. (1997) *Dementia Reconsidered: The Person Comes First.* Buckingham: Open University Press.

Lewis, F. (July 2015) *Estimation of future cases of dementia from those born in 2015.* Consultation report for Alzheimer's Research UK.

Mahoney, R., Regan, C., Katona, C. and Livingston, G. (2005) "Anxiety and Depression in Family Caregivers of People with Alzheimer's Disease: the LASER-AD Study." *American Jouranal of Geriatric Psychiatry*, 13 (9), 795–801.

Maslow, A. H. (1943) "A theory of human motivation." *Psychological Review*, 50(4), 370–396.

National Institute on Aging (n.d.) Safe Use of Medicines for Older Adults. Available at www.nia.nih.gov/health/safe-use-medicines-older-adults

National Institute on Aging (n.d.) Choosing Healthy Meals As You Get Older. Available at www.nia.nih.gov/health/healthy-eating

Prince, M *et al.* (2014) *Dementia UK: Update.* Second edition. Report produced by King's College London and the London School of Economics for the Alzheimer's Society.

Tulving, E. (1985) Memory and consciousness. *Canadian Psychology/Psychologie Canadienne,* 26(1), 1–12.

INDEX

Sub-headings in *italics* indicate figures.

acceptance 98
activity 84, 141
   activity loss 50
   daily living 123–5
   environment 125–7
   motor function 99–100
   personal care 121–3
Alzheimer's disease 19, 20, 90
   amnesic Alzheimer's disease 20
   atypical Alzheimer's disease 21
   dysexecutive Alzheimer's disease 22
   lopogenic progressive aphasia 21
   posterior cortical atrophy (PCA) 21
   retrieving a memory 90, 91
   symptoms of amnesic Alzheimer's disease 22–4
Alzheimer's Research UK 12
Alzheimer's Society Dementia UK Report 12
anger 98
anosagnosia 97
Antecedent Behaviour Consequence (ABC) charts 69–71
anxiety 108–9
apraxia 99
ataxia 99
Atkinson, R. C. 167
attention 88–9
awareness 97
  acceptance 98
  anger 98
  denial 97
  depression 98
  unawareness 97
  uncertainty 97–8

behaviour 57
   behaviour and personality changes 99
   behaviour as communication 61–3
   Behaviour Record Charts 69, 72–4, 143, 144
   John's story 59–61, 71
   Margaret 147–58
   Margaret's behaviour problems 149–50
   Margaret's Behaviour Record Charts 150–2, 157, 158
   perspective 63–7
   Sally's story 57–9
   Susan's story 58
behavioural variant frontotemporal dementia 30–1
brain 14–15
   brain diseases 14
   frontal lobe 15–17
   occipital lobe 18
   parietal lobe 17
   temporal lobe 17–18

carers 131, 133, 138–9
   explaining the behaviour of the person with dementia 145
   family and friends who are carers 134–6
   Fred and Sadie 136–8

carers *cont.*
   helping carers to understand when behaviours occur 143
   Initial Contact form 144, 150
   life history of person with dementia 145
   meeting with staff and carers 146
   paid carers 139–40
   Review document 144
   sharing information with care home staff 143
   Understanding document 144, 146
   what might help address unmet need 145
CLEAR Dementia Care© 62, 65, 79, 140, 141–2, 158
   assessment 140, 145
   Behaviour Record Charts 69, 72–4, 143, 144
   CLEAR Dementia Care© Model 84, 142
   five domains 83–4
   Initial Contact form 143, 144, 150
   Medication Record Charts 143
   Review document 143, 144
   Understanding document 106–7, 144, 146
cognition 83, 85, 141
   attention and concentration 88–9
   awareness 97–8
   behaviour and personality changes 99
   delusions 100
   driving 101
   executive function 95–6
   hallucinations 100
   illusions 100
   language 92–4
   memory 89–92
   motor function 99–100
   orientation 85–7
   sleep disturbances 101
   speed of processing 87–8
   visuospatial processing 94–5
concentration 88–9
constipation 117–18
coping strategies 109
corticobasal syndrome (CBS) 33–4

dehydration 116
   prevention 117
   symptoms 117
delirium 112–13
   offering care 115–16
   symptoms 113–14
   types of delirium 115
delusions 100
dementia 11–13, 19
   Alzheimer's disease 19, 20–4
   frontotemporal dementia (FTD) 19, 30–5

   hierarchy of needs theory 76–9
   Lewy body dementia 19, 27–9
   Mary's story 12–13
   mixed dementia 19, 36
   other dementias 19, 36
   unrelated conditions affecting memory 14
   vascular dementia 19, 24–7
denial 97
depression 14, 98, 107
   symptoms 108
   what can you do to help? 108
disorientation 95
driving 101
drunkenness 14
Duffy, F. 62, 143
dysexecutive Alzheimer's disease 22

emotional wellbeing 84, 107–10, 141
   anxiety 108–9
   controlling emotions 109
   coping strategies 109
   depression 107–8
   previous mental health difficulties 109
environment 84, 125–6
   changes to the environment 126–7
executive function 95–6

frontotemporal dementia (FTD) 19, 30
   behavioural variant frontotemporal dementia 30–1
   motor variant frontotemporal dementia 33–5
   primary progressive aphasia 31–2
   types of frontotemporal dementia 30

hallucinations 100
head injuries 14
hearing loss 119–20
home loss 46–8
hyperactive delirium 115
hypoactive delirium 115

illusions 100
incontinence 121
independence loss 49–50
infections 112
Initial Contact form 143, 144, 150

James, I. A. 69

kidney disorders 14
Kitwood, T. 63, 71

INDEX

language 92–4
Lewis, F. 12
Lewy body dementia 19, 27
    symptoms 27–9
life story 83, 141, 145
    Anna 106
    Brenda 104–5
    Kate 103
    Life Story books 107
    Michael 105–6
    personality 101–2
    Robert 105
    Understanding document 106–7, 144, 146
liver disorders 14
long-term health conditions 120–1
long-term memory 92
lopogenic progressive aphasia 21
loss 37–9
    loss of activity 50
    loss of familiar routines 49
    loss of home 46–8
    loss of independence 49–50
    loss of memory 39–41
    loss of relationship 43–6
    loss of role 41–2
    loss of social contact 42–3
    sensory impairment 119–20

Mahoney, R. 135
Maslow, A. H. 75–6
medications 118
    Medication Record Charts 143
    medication side effects 14
memory 89
    encoding information into memory 89
    memory loss 39–41
    retrieving a memory 90–1
    storing information as a memory 89–90
    types of memory 91–2
mixed delirium 115
mixed dementia 19, 36
motor function 99–100
motor neurone disease (MND) 35
motor variant frontotemporal dementia 33–5
multi-infarct dementia 25

National Institute on Aging 14
needs 75–9
    Maslow's Hierarchy of Needs 75
Newcastle model 69
nutritional deficiencies 14

orientation 85
    orientation to person 87
    orientation to place 86–7
    orientation to time 85–6

pain 110, 143
    how do we respond to pain? 111–12
    long-term conditions that can cause pain 111
    short-term conditions that can cause pain 110–11
peripheral vision 95
personality 83, 101–2
    behaviour and personality changes 99
    life story and personality 103–7
physical wellbeing 84, 110
    constipation 117–18
    dehydration 116–17
    delirium 112–16
    infections 112
    long-term health conditions 120–1
    medications 118
    pain 110–12
    sensory impairment 119–20
posterior cortical atrophy (PCA) 21
primary progressive aphasia 31–2
Prince, M. 12, 19, 20, 24, 27, 30
procedural memory 92
processing speed 87–8
progressive non-fluent aphasia 32
progressive supranuclear palsy (PSP) 34–5

reading 94, 95
relationships 84, 128–9, 141
    carers 131
    family and friends 130
    other residents 131–2
    relationship loss 43–6
    safety in relationships 132
REM Sleep Disorder 29, 101
respiratory infections 112
Review document 143, 144
Richardson, J. 62, 143
role loss 41–2
routine loss 49

self 51–6
semantic dementia 31–2
semantic memory 92
sensory impairment 119
    dementia and hearing loss 120
    dementia and sight loss 120
Shiffrin, R. M. 91

short-term memory 91
sight loss 119–20
sleep disturbance 14, 101
SMART (Specific, Measurable, Achievable, Realistic and Time-scaled) recommendations 146
social contact loss 42–3
stigma 78–9
stroke-related dementia 25
sub-cortical vascular dementia 25

thyroid disorders 14
Tulving, E. 91

unawareness 97
uncertainty 97–8
Understanding document 106–7, 144, 146
urinary tract infections (UTIs) 112

vascular dementia 19, 24
 retrieving a memory 90–1
 stroke-related or multi-infarct dementia 25
 sub-cortical vascular dementia 25
 symptoms 25–7
visuospatial processing 94–5

writing 94